HOMEOPATHY
A COMPARATIVE MATERIA MEDICA

In a healthy
man, the vital force
keeps the entire organism
in harmonious order. In a diseased
man, this vital force is deranged and this
derangement expresses itself by abnormal
sensations and functions of the
organism. These sensations,
or disease signs, are
called disease
symptoms.
In Homoeopathy,
there is no disease named
like Influenza or Typhoid, but a
sum total of the symptoms of a disease.
This totality of symptoms is the
only guide to the selection
of a remedy.

HOMEOPATHY
A Comparative Materia Medica

(Part I)

S. Kumar

New Age Books

ISBN: 81-7822-040-7 (2 Pts.)

First Edition: **Delhi, 2005**

Published by
NEW AGE BOOKS
A-44 Naraina Phase I
New Delhi-110 028 (INDIA)
Email: nab@vsnl.in
Website: www.newagebooksindia.com

Printed in India
at Shri Jainendra Press
A-45 Naraina Phase-I, New Delhi-110 028

To
my father
who wanted to
see this book in print

CONTENTS

Foreword xiii
Preface xv
Acknowledgements xvii
Rubricks xviii

Part I

Towards Understanding Homeopathy 3
Aconitum Napellus 9
Actaea Recemosa 15
Aesculus Hippocastanum 17
Athusa Cynapium 21
Agaricus Muscarius 23
Allium Cepa 27
Aloe Soccotrina 29
Alumina 31
Ammonium Carbonicum 35
Ammonium Muriaticum 39
Amylenum Nitrosum 41
Anacardium Orintale 43
Antimonium Crudum 47
Antimonium Tartaricum 53
Apis Mellifica 59
Argentum Metallicum 63
Argentum Nitricum 65
Arnica Montana 69
Arsenicum Album 75
Arum Triphyllum 83
Asafoetida 85
Aurum Metallicum 87
Baptisia Tinctoria 91
Baryta Carbonica 95
Belladonna 97
Benzoic Acid 105

Berberis Vulgaris	107
Bismuth	109
Borax	111
Bromium	115
Bryonia Alba	119
Cactus Grandiflorus	127
Calcarea Carbonica	131
Calcarea Phosphorica	143
Camphora	147
Cannabis Indica	151
Cannabis Sativa	155
Cantheris	157
Capsicum	161
Carbo Animalis	167
Carbo Vegetabilis	169
Caulophyllum	175
Causticum	177
Chamomilla	187
Chelidonium Majus	197
Chenopodium	203
Chimaphilla	205
China	207
Cicuta Virosa	211
Cimicifuga	215
Cina	217
Clematis	221
Cocculus	223
Coffea Cruda	231
Colchicum Autumnale	235
Collinsonia Canadensis	239
Colocynthis	241
Conium Maculatum	245
Copaiva	251
Corallium	253
Crocus Sativus	255
Crotalus Horridus	257
Croton Tiglium	259
Cuprum Metallicum	261
Digitalis Purpurea	263

Dioscorea Villosa 267
Drosera Rotundifolia 269
Dulcamara 273
Equisetum Hyemale 277
Eupatorium Perfoliatum 279
Euphrasia 281
Ferrum Metallicum 283
Ferrum Phosphoricum 289
Fluoric Acid 291
Gelsemium 293
Glonoine 299
Graphites 303
Hamamelis Virginica 309
Helleborus Niger 311
Hepar Sulphuris 313
Hydrastis Canadensis 319
Hyoscyamus Niger 321
Ignatia 327
Iodium 335
Ipecacuanha 339
Iris Versicolor 345
Kali Salts 347
Kali Bromatum 349
Kali Carbonicum 353
Kali Iodatum 359
Kali Sulphuricum 361
Kalmia Latifolia 363
Kreosotum 365
Lac Caninum 369
Lachesis 373
Ledum Palustre 381
Lilium Tigrinum 387
Lobelia Inflata 391
Lycopodium Clavatum 393
Magnesia Carbonica 403
Magnesia Muriatica 405
Magnesia Phosphorica 407
Medorrhinum 411

Part II

Melilotus Alba	415
Mercurius Corrosivus	417
Mercurius Cyanatus	421
Mercurius Solubilis	423
Mezereum	431
Millefolium	435
Murex Purpurea	437
Muriatic Acid	439
Naja Tripudians	443
Natrum Arsenicum	445
Natrum Carbonicum	447
Natrum Muriaticum	449
Natrum Phosphoricum	459
Natrum Sulphuricum	461
Nitric Acidum	465
Nux Moschata	473
Nux Vomica	479
Opium	489
Petroleum	493
Petroselinum	497
Phosphoric-acid	499
Phosphorus	505
Phytolacca	513
Platinum	517
Plumbum	521
Psorinum	525
Pulsatilla	529
Rheum	537
Rhododendron	539
Rhus Toxicodendron	541
Rumex Crispus	549
Ruta Graveolens	551
Sabadilla	557
Sabina	559
Sambucus Nigra	561
Sanguinaria	563
Sanicula	567
Sarsaparilla	569

Secale Cornutum 573
Selenium 577
Sepia 579
Silicea 587
Spigelia 595
Spongia Tosta 597
Stannum 599
Staphisagria 603
Sticta Pulmonaria 611
Sulphur 613
Sulphuric Acid 625
Tabacum 629
Tarentula 631
Terebinthina 635
Theridion Curassavicum 639
Thuja Occidentalis 641
Trillium Pendulum 645
Tuberculinum Bacillinum 647
Valeriana 649
Veratrum Album 651
Veratrum Viride 657
Viburnum Opulus 659
Zincum 661

List of Remedies 665
Glossary of Medical Terms 673
Understanding Homeopathic Medicines 709
Index of Medicines 717
Index of Diseases and Symptoms 729

Foreword

I know personally the author as a good Homeopath for the last seventeen years. I had the opportunity of meeting Shri Santosh Kumar, ADG of Police, at the end of the year 1978 and since then the acquaintance strengthened. He has keen interest in Homeopathy. He has treated so many patients voluntarily to carry out his mission.

His long, rich experience is now reduced in writing. This book he has written will be a source of inspiration to all those who follow the path shown by the author and I am sure the book will be very helpful to the students, teachers of Homeopathy and practitioners for ready reference.

Regd. No. 2531 (Bihar)
Patel Nagar, Patna-23

—Dr. B. Bhattacharya
Ex-Chairman
State Board of Homeopathic Medicine
Bihar, India,
Ex-Chairman, All India Homeopathic
Medical Association of India 1983-85;
Ex-Chairman, Bidya Vati Girls' School, Patna, Bihar;
Life Member, Bihar Hindi Sahitya Sammelan, Patna, Bihar

Preface

I had read somewhere that every Homeopath writes his own Materia Medica. To me that is why, we have so many books every year on homeopathy including mine. If everyone could be satisfied with set principles alone, without critically examining, expending them, then there would have been very few books on shelf of world library. But a principle once fixed remains static—but time, circumstances, and human experience with that principle in particular goes on enhancing—resulting in analysis of the principle, expansion, new dimensions and new explanations. This goes on and new books come in on.

Homeopathy is rarely, the first choice for treatment. I was no exception. Our daughter was few days old, she was very thin, weak and delicate. When she contacted her first infection. Mr. S.N. Puri, a very close friend, advised us to show her to him. Dr. Bhattacharya prescribed her some medicines. I was anxious to know what was given. He sensed my anxiety and advised me that I should look about those medicines in a homeopathic book called Materia Medica by Boericke. I went through the medicines. Curiously I read further. On next appointment, I discussed what I had read. He encouraged me and thus he put me on road to Homeopathy.

After reading a few books, I started noticing, to get a fuller picture of a drug. Cowperthwate introduced a medicine and its action on a healthy body well. Allen's book especially described constitutions of the patient. Nash's book compared drugs and common symptoms diligently. Dr. Bhattacharya also permitted me to sit with him from time to time in his chamber, to watch how he examined patients and prescribed medicines. I observed there how disease symptoms were matched with medicine-symptoms. Then it occurred why not put all these leading characteristics found in different books together.

This all gradually lead me to compile these characteristics of a medicine. I wrote up a few medicines and showed them to Dr. Bhattacharya. He encouraged to add more characteristics and medicines. Gradually it became a lengthy compilation in the present form.

Most time taking to grasp was that the Homeopathy cures the patient, not the disease. Then it became clear what was meant by "1000 medicines—one disease, 1000 diseases, one medicine. The three constitutional miasmas remind us three Tridosh—Vata, pitta, kapha—of our own system of medicine, Ayurveda (Knowledge of long life). It may not be ruled out that Indian Tridosh had reached Germany before Hahnemann, because many Sanskrit masterpieces had already been translated in German before the time of Hahnemann. Whatever the facts may be but Homeopathy miasmas and Ayurvedic Tridosh resemble closely.

Though, thorough care has been taken to mimimize the mistakes in the book, but there must have crept in some. As mistakes in other books hurt my eyes, mine will do the same to others. I seek indulgence and pardon.

If it helps in curing even one person my effort will be amply rewarded.

S. KUMAR

Acknowledgements

I AM INDEBTED TO:

• My Guru, friend and philosopher Dr. B. Bhattacharya for leading me on path of Homeopathy, his unbound faith in me, for insights and constantly prodding to complete this book.

• To my father who much looked forward to see this book in print but could not.

• Shri S.N. Puri, my well wisher and elder brother, who introduced me to Dr. B. Bhattacharya.

• All Masters of Homeopathy, from whose genius, I have borrowed, extracted, and culled.

• Shri Anil Kumar, who first typed the tedious manuscript, Sri Krishna Nand who freshly typed and prepared final copy, Sri Kumar Anand Mohan, who put this lengthly book on a floppy.

• Krishna Chaudhary, my friend and colleague, who computerized the book again, prepared indices, read entire book corrected and improved both language and grammar. His deep knowledge of silviculture, helped me to understand many plant medicines better. Without him the book would have remained a poorer version.

• Shri Kamala Shankar Singh, who of his own talked to the proprietors of New Age Books about this book.

• Shri J.P. Jain who asked for the manuscript, then suggested some improvements, and accepted for publication, in a very short time.

• Shri Rajeev Jain for accepting this book for his new venture and making such an excellent job in very short time.

• Last but not the least my wife and daughter had to suffer many medicines, many times, sometimes willingly, and our pet Tipsy every time forcibly.

S. Kumar

Arrangement of Rubricks

The following arrangement has been followed uniformly in the book while describing a medicine. Exceptions, if any, have been mentioned wherever they occur:

1. Introduction	-Cowperth waite, 1984 (B. Jain, N. Delhi)
2. General Analysis	-Cowperth waite, 1984 (B. Jain, N. Delhi)
3. Suited to	-Allen's Key Note, 1977 (Calcutta).
4. Clinical particulars	-Clarke's Dictionary of Materia Medica Vols. I, II and III
5. General Symptoms	-Nash, (Leaders, New Delhi)
6. Particular Symptoms	-Nash, (Leaders, New Delhi)
7. Black Letter Symptoms	-Tyler, Drug Pictures, 1975 (N. Delhi)
8. Plain Talks on Materia Medica	-Pierce W.I.
9. Chronic Diseases	-Hahnemann, New Delhi
10. Materia Medica Pura	-Hahnemann, New Delhi
11. Organon of Medicine	-Hahnemann, New Delhi
12. Farrington's Materia Medica	-8th Edition, Calcutta
13. Principles and Practice of Homeopathy	-Richard Hughes

HOMEOPATHY
A Comparative Materia Medica

(Part I)

TOWARDS UNDERSTANDING HOMEOPATHY

(Organon of Medicine)

Like all epoch making discoveries in the world, Homeopathy was also a chance discovery by Dr. Samuel Hahnemann, an allopath. It was a new system of attending to the disease, or to be more exact, the patient, or attending to the curable in the disease. He explained and laid down the main principles of his system in a book called "Organon of medicine".

The main principles of the Organon are as follows:

The sole aim of the physician (Homeopath) is to cure the patient rapidly, gently, and permanently. To achieve this aim he must find out what is curable in the disease and what is curative in medicine. In a healthy man, vital force keeps the entire organism in harmonious order. In a diseased man, this vital force in him is deranged and this derangement expresses itself by abnormal sensations and functions of the organism. These sensations, or disease signs, are called disease symptoms. For the physician, the disease means the totality of its symptoms. He needs only to take away this totality of symptoms to take away the entire disease.

In simple words, it means that in Homeopathy there is no disease name like Influenza or Typhoid, but a sum total of the symptoms of a disease, the name of the disease notwithstanding. This totality of symptoms is the only guide to the selection of a remedy which leads to rapid, gentle and permanent cure.

Disease and Medicine

Medicine has the power of producing alterations in a healthy man's health. If a medicine does not alter a healthy man's health, and does not produce abnormal sensations and functions in the organism, it does not have the power to cure. This power can only be ascertained by its effects on healthy persons. The morbid symptoms that medicines produce in healthy persons are the only symptoms the medicines can cure. That is the disease curing power of the medicine.

The curative power of medicines therefore depends on the symptoms they have which are similar to the ***disease***. "***Similia similibus curentur***", *i.e.*, similar cures similar. The symptoms which a medicine produces in a healthy man, it cures in a diseased man.

Action of Medicine

Every medicine has two actions, one primary and the other secondary. The primary action takes place under the influence of every medicine, and the secondary action or reaction is affected in the living organism. To illustrate this—when a healthy man takes a medicine, its primary action produces disease symptoms in the healthy man. When a .diseased person having similar symptoms takes the same medicine, then the secondary action is affected by the diseased organism and this secondary action leads to cure.

Three steps are necessary for cure:

1. Investigation of the disease—what can be cured in a disease.
2. Investigation of the effects of a medicine on healthy persons to obtain the disease signs which it can cure.
3. Appropriate application of the medicine—matching the symptoms of the medicine to the symptoms of the disease. The medicine most close to the disease symptoms will effect the cure.

Chronic and Acute Diseases

Diseases have been classified as: (1) Acute, and (2) Chronic.

Diseases which have a tendency to finish their course more or less quickly, but always in a moderate time, are known as acute diseases. Chronic diseases have often imperceptible beginnings. They derange the living organism, and gradually cause it to deviate from its healthy condition in such a way that automatic life energy, the vital force, opposes such diseases only at the commencement, and during their progress offers helpless and useless resistance. Then the organism helplessly suffers from them. The diseases go on increasing their morbid influence upon the organism, destroying it in the end. A chronic miasma causes these diseases and they are the most incurable.

Chronic Miasma

During his experience as a homeopath Hahnemann noticed that in some cases even the best selected medicines ensured only temporary relief instead of permanent cure. With careful, critical and analytical study he concluded that there was morbid force between the curative power of the medicine and the curable in the disease which did not allow the action of the medicine to run its full course. He called this force Miasma and identified three such distinct forces: (1) Syphilis, (2) Sycosis and (3) Psora. Syphilis was known to some extent from before as a chronic disease.

Sycosis [Condylomatus (Tumour, warts, or late secondary syphilis manifestation in and around genitals) disease], inirradicable by the vital force without proper medicinal treatment was not recognised as a chronic miasmatic disease. Physicians believed that they had cured the disease when they had destroyed the growth upon the skin but its persistent dyscrasia (morbid state resulting from toxic materials in the blood) escaped their observation. Psora, Hahnemann found after twelve years of investigation, was the mother of all chronic diseases except Syphilis and Sycosis, and responsible for most of the chronic diseases.

While the other two reveal their specific internal toxic material (dyscrasia)—Syphilis by venereal chancre (the primary sphletic ulcer), and Sycosis by the cauliflower-like growths—Psora announces itself by a peculiar cutaneous (relating to the skin) eruption, sometimes consisting of only a few vesicles, accompanied by intolerable voluptuous tickling itching with a peculiar odour. Psora produces numerous other forms of disease ranging from nervous debility to urinary Calculi.

Medicinal Investigation

The process of administration of a medicine to a healthy man, and collation of the symptoms which develop on the healthy organism, is called "proving" of the medicine which demonstrates the pure effects of the medicine. The action of every medicine differs from every other medicine.

Employment of the Medicine

The medicine most homoeopathically corresponding is the most suitable, the most specific. Homeopathic means that the pure effects of the medicine match most suitably the symptoms of the disease in an individual.

Epidemics

The same Homeopathic principle applies to epidemics. It must be understood that all those who are affected by the prevailing epidemic have certainly contracted it from the same source and, hence, are suffering from the same disease. However, the whole extent of the epidemic disease cannot be learned from one patient or two but from several patients with different constitutions. Then the area suffering becomes one single patient, and common symptoms the disease signs.

Single Medicine

Only one single simple medicine should be given to the patient at one time (274-u). Of late, combination of several medicines, are quite in vogue, though they donot conform to this rule.

The medicine should be stopped as soon as improvement sets in. This applies to both acute and chronic diseases (246).

It is impractical to repeat the same dose of a medicine. The succeeding dose should be slightly strengthened by shaking the bottle before giving the dose (note to 247).

Signs of Improvement

The patient complains of no new symptoms and old symptoms are not worse. Besides, if an improvement in the disposition and mind has been observed, then the medicine has effected positive diminution of the disease (255).

In acute diseases, a slight commencement of amelioration or aggravation, the state of mind of the patient and his whole demeanour are informative. In case of slight improvement a greater degree of comfort, calmness, freedom of mind, higher spirits—a kind of return of the natural state is observed. In case of small aggravation the exact opposite is observed (253).

Note: Brackets indicate rules of the Organon.

ACONITUM NAPELLUS

I. Introduction (Cow-9)

Synonym: Aconitum Napellus.
Natural Order: Ranunculaceæ.
Common Name: Monk's Hood.
Habitat: Europe, America (cultivated).
Preparation: Tincture of the whole plant, gathered at the time of flowering. It was proved by Hahnemann and his disciples. (MMP records 540 symptoms). He used it in the dose of a 1000th part of a drop of the decillionth development of power (MMP IIIrd Ed. pg.-25).

II. General Analysis (Cow)

Acts mainly upon cerebrospinal system producing exalted activity in arterial circulation; congestion and inflammation of various parts of the body. There is very little evidence that Acon. produces any organic changes. Its leading expression is—Feverish, nervous, restlessness or mental distress, full pounding pulse.

III. Suited to (Allen-15)

Acute or recent cases in young persons, esp. girls of a full plethoric habit, of sedentary life; persons easily affected by atmospheric changes; of rigid muscular fibre < dark hair and eyes.

IV. Clinical (Clarke-I-15)

Amaurosis, Anger, Apoplexy, Asthma, Blindness-sudden, Bronchitis, Catalepsy, Catheter fever, Chestaffections of, Chickenpox, Cholera, Cholera infantum, Colds, Coldness, Consumption, Convulsions, Cough, Croup, Cystitis, Dengue fever, Dentition, Diarrhoea, Dropsy, Dysentery, Dysmenorrhoea, Ear affections, Enteritis, Erythema nodosum,

Excitement, Eye affections, Face-flushing of, Fever-effects of, Fever, Fear-effects of, Glands swollen, Glossitis, Gonorrhoea, Haemorrhage, Haemorrhoids-strangulated, Headache, Heart affections, Hip-joint disease, Hodgkin's disease, Hyperpyrexia, Influenza, Jaundice, Joint affections, Labour, Lactation, Laryngitis, Liver-inflammation of, Lumbago, Lung affections, Mania, Measles, Meningitis, Menstruation disordered, Miliaria, Miscarriage, Mumps, Myalgia, Myelitis, Nephritis, Neuralgia, Numbness, Oesophagus-inflammation of, Paralysis, Peritonitis, Phlegmasia alba dolens, Pleurisy, Pleurodynia, Pneumonia, Pregnancy, Puerperal fever, Purpura, Quinsy, Remittent fever, Roseola, Scarlatina, Shivering, Sleeplessness, Smell disordered, Stiff-neck, Testicles-affections of, Tetanus, Tetany, Thirst, Throat-affections of, Tongue-affections of, Toothache, Traumatic fever, Urethra-spasmodic stricture of, Urethral fever, Urine-suppression of, Uterus-prolapse of, Vaccination-effects of, Vertigo, Whooping-cough, Yawning, Yellow fever.

V. Symptoms-General (Nash-82)

1. Fear of death, of crowds, of going out, Anything-always fearful.
2. Complaints from exposure to cold, dry cold.
3. Congestion and inflammation, acute, first stage with great anxiety, heat and restlessness; tosses about in agony; throws off covering.
4. Inflammatory fever.
5. Pains insuppressable, < at night, especially in the evening, neuralgic.
6. Face very red and flushed, but turns pale on rising up.
7. Favourite points of attack-Larynx (Croup), Bronchi (Bronchitis), Lungs and Pleura (Pneumonia and Pleurisy), Joints (Rheumatism), heart and Circulation (Erethism).
8. Modalities < In the evening (Chest symptoms and pains), Lying on left side; in warm room or warm covering.
9. > Uncovering-Kicks the clothes off.

VI. Symptoms-Particular (Nash-82)

Symptom	Remedy	Characteristics
(a) Restlessness (Trio)	Acon.	—Pain cutting tearing. Early stage.
		—Fear of death **(Leading Characteristic)** almost always present.
	Ars.	—with extreme weakness, wants to move from place to place but is not relieved.
		—Later stage, restlessness.
	Rhus t.	—Aching Pains which make him move for temporary relief which he gets from movement which Acon., and Ars., don't get.
		—With numbness, soreness (dull and aching).
(b) Inflammatory Affections	Acon.	—Dry, hot skin, no sweat
	Bell.	—Greater hot skin but sweat on covered parts.
(Acon. = Bell.)	Acon.	—Tosses in agony with great fear of death.
	Bell.	—Semi stupor, jerks and twitches in sleep.
	Acon.	—Great distress, in heart and chest.
	Bell.	—Everything seems to centre in the head.
	Acon.	—Fears death.
	Bell.	—Fears things imaginary with delirium.
(c) Pain	Acon.	
	Cham.	
	Coff.	
	Rhus t.	
(d) Painlessness	Op., Stram.	
(e) Fright (either immediate or remote)	Acon.	
	Op.	
	Ign.	
	Verat.	

(f) Dry-Cold Air < Acon. -(19 out of 20 Croups covered by it).
Bry.
Caust.
Hep. s.
Nux. v.

(g) Wet air remedies < Dulc.
Nux. m.
Nat. s.
Rhus t.

VII. Black Letter Symptoms (Tyler-8-11)

- Nightly raging delirium.
- Variable humour-gay, then dejected.
- He did all things hurriedly.
- Great vexation about trifles.
- Great anxiety; great internal anxiety.
- Inconsolable anxiety.
- Extremely disposed to be cross.
- Fear of approaching death.
- Lamentable fears of approaching death.
- Apprehension; Sadness; Solicitude.
- Fear of some misfortune happening to him.
- Inconsolable anxiety and piteous howling, with complaints and reproaches about (often trivial) evils.
- Excessive restlessness and tossing about for hours.
- Mental—very restless nights. Restless tossing in bed.
- Palpitation of heart and great anxiety; increased heat of body, especially in the face. She is as if stupefied from flying redness in the face.
- Unsteadiness of ideas—if she wants to pursue a train of thought, a second chases this away, and a third again displaces this, until she become quite confused.
- Want of memory, as if what he had just done were a dream, and he can scarcely recall what it was.
- Weakness of memory.
- HEAD in front as if nailed up.
- Pain is intolerable, drives him crazy.

- Fullness and heaviness in forehead as if an out-pressing weight lay there and as if all would be forced out at the forehead.
- Heat in head. Burning headache as if brain agitated by boiling water.
- Fullness in head. Semilateral drawing in head.
- Throbbing left side forehead, while strong beats occur in right side by fits.
- Vertigo: staggers especially to the right.
- Vertigo with nausea, especially rising from sitting.
- Vertigo worse shaking head, whereby complete darkness comes before eyes.
- Dilated pupils. Photophobia.
- Inflammation EYES with lachrymation, which causes so much pain and fright that he wishes for death.
- Inflammation of eyes, extremely painful.
- Great sensitivity to NOISE.
- EPISTAXIS.
- Great sensitivity of olfactory nerve.
- Creeping pain in CHEEKS.
- Sensation of the face growing large.
- Penetrating fine stitches in tip of TONGUE.
- Tongue swollen
- Dryness of mouth.
- Burning in THROAT.
- Great thirst.
- Empty Eructation. Nausea.
- Vomits lumbrici.
- Inclination to vomit as if had eaten something disgustingly sweet/greasy.
- Violent vomiting.
- Pressive pain, STOMACH, like a weight
- Tensive pressing pain, like a weight in stomach and hypochondria.
- Swollen, distended ABDOMEN, like ascites.
- Flatulent colic in hypo-gastrium as if he had taken a flatus-producing purgative.
- Burning in umbilical region.
- Sensitivity of abdomen to touch, as from slight peritoneal inflammation.

- Burning in abdomen.
- Cutting in intestines.
- Great swelling of abdomen which is painful to touch.
- White STOOL.
- Pain in rectum, shooting and aching in anus.
- Anxious desire to urinate.
- URINE hot dark coloured.
- Foetid breath.
- Sensitiveness of LARYNX to touch.
- Hoarseness. Hoarse, dry, loud cough.
- Expectoration of bright red blood. Haemoptysis.
- Difficult respiration.
- Squeezing pain in chest.
- Creeping pain in chest. Stitches in chest with cough.
- Anxiety about HEART. Palpitation and anxiety.
- Pulse contracted, full powerful, febrile, exceeding 100 beats to a minute.
- Rheumatic pain, nape of NECK-only on moving
- Violent, shooting, digging pain left of spine.
- Bruised pain in articulation of lowest lumbar vertebra with sacrum: feels hacked off.
- Cool sweat on PALMS.
- Creeping pain in fingers.
- Coldness of feet.
- Weakness and laxity of the ligaments of all joints.
- Yawns often without being sleepy.
- Light SLEEP.
- Very restless nights: tossing in bed. Excessive restlessness.
- Anxious dreams: wakes with a start.
- Chill of whole body with hot forehead: hot ear and internal, dry heat.
- Slight perspiration all over body.
- Very fine stinging, or stinging burning pain in many parts, skin.
- Redness and heat of one, coldness and paleness of the other cheek.
- Towards evening, burning heat in head and face, redness of cheeks and out-pressing headache.
- Towards evening, dry heat in face with anxiety.

ACTAEA RECEMOSA

I. Suited to (Allen-17)

Woman who thinks she is going crazy. (Syph.) illusion of mouse running under her chair (Lach., Aeth. c.), puerperal mania, sensation as if a heavy, black cloud had settled all over her.

II. Clinical (Clarke-I-25)

Abortion-tendency to, Angina pectoris, Appetite disordered, Back pains, Breasts-affection of, Cerebro-spinal meningitis, Change of life, Chest-pains in, Chorea, Delirium tremens, Diaphragm-rheumatism of, Dyspepsia, Epilepsy. Faintness, Headache, Heart affections, Hyperpyrexia, Hypochondriasis, Hysteria, Lumbago, Melancholia, Meningitis, Menstruation disordered, Myalgia, Neuralgia, Ovaries-affections of, Perichondritis, Pleurodynia, Pregnancy-affections of, Puerperal mania, Rheumatic gout, Rheumatism, Sciatica, Side pain, Sinking sensation, Sleeplessness, Spinal irritation, Stiff-neck, Tinnitus aurium, Tremors, Uterine affections, Vomiting of pregnancy.

III. Symptoms-General (Nash-214)

1. Nervous symptoms, twitchings, spasms, Convulsion, neuralgias; chills without shaking; < at menstrual period.
2. Muscular rheumatism; stiff neck, drawing head back; can't turn the head; rheumatism of the belly of muscles, by preference.
3. Headaches; pressing outward; or upward, as if top of head would fly off, or in to eyes (Ciliary neuralgia), or down nape into spine.
4. Gloomy, sad, sleepless; thinks she will go insane.

5. Menorrhagia; pains run through hips into thighs, passing down.
6. Climacteric; infra-mammary pains left side, persistent.
7. Modalities < menstrual period and during climacteric.

IV. **Symptoms-Particular** (Nash-215-16)

1. Very gloomy with sleeplessness. Nervous chill without coldness; faints; talks incessantly, frequently changing subjects; is grieved and troubled.
2. Severe headache pressing outward, running into eyes which ache fearfully; pain settles down in the occiput and shoots down the neck.
   Almost specific for Ciliary neuralgia.
3. One of the best remedies in Menorrhagia with "severe pain in back down to thighs", "Pain in the uterine region, darting from side to side".
4. Infra-mammary pain in the left side during climacteric.
5. Backache, spinal irritation, sharp lancinating pains, in various parts, nervous or muscular. } With uterine disturbances
6. Rheumatic affection attacks belly of muscle by preference.

AESCULUS HIPPOCASTANUM

I. Introduction (Cow-19)

Natural Order: Sapindacæ.
Common Name: Horse chest-nut.
Habitat: A tree native to middle Asia but cultivated in temperate climate.
Preparation: Tincture from fresh ripe hulled nut.

II. General Analysis (Cow)

Acts mainly upon the liver and portal system, causing congestion, secondarily giving rise to *catarhal inflammation in the colon, rectum and anus; intense congestion of haemorrhoidal vessels.* Chief characteristic—severe aching pain in lumber and sacral regions.

III. Suited to (Allen-19)

Persons with haemorrhoidal tendencies and who suffer with Gastric, Bilious, or Catarrhal troubles; Fullness in various parts (as from an undue amount of blood)—heart, lung, stomach, brain, anus etc.

IV. Clinical (Clarke-I-32)

Anus-affections of, Back-affections of, Constipation, Cough, Haemorrhoids, Headache, Hernia, Intermittents, Jaundice, Liver-affections of, Lumbago, Prostate-affections of, Sacrum-pain in, Taste disordered, Throat-affections of, Tongue-affections of, Uterus-prolapse of.

V. Symptoms-General (Nash-179)

1. Sense of fullness and pulsation in various organs and veins (especially plethoric), as if too full of blood.
2. Constant dull backache across sacrum and hips; <

walking or on stooping (piles, leucorrhoea, displacements, etc.).

3. Sense of fullness, as of sticks in the rectum (Haemorrhoids).
4. Mucous membranes of mouth, throat, rectum are swollen, burn, dry and raw.
5. Coryza; thin, watery, burning; rawness and sensitivity to inhaled cold air.
6. Frequent inclination to swallow, with burning, pricking, stinging and dry constricted fauces (Apis., Bell.)

VI. Symptoms-Particular (Nash-180)

Almost all its usefulness centres in its action in the lower back and pelvic region—"constant dull Backache much < stooping or walking".

1. One of the leading remedies for haemorrhoids and backache. There is a feeling of "fullness, dryness" and sticking as if rectum was full of sticks, without tendency to protrusion or prolapsus, which is in Ign., Aloe., Podo., and the backache greatly out of proportion.
2. These symptoms are found in conjunction with other affections such as uterus displacements and inflammations and some very bad forms of leucorrhoea.
3. Throbbing or beating sensations are another valuable symptom.
4. Coryza-like Ars. but with sensation of rawness, sensitive to inhaled cold air. Same rawness in throat.

VII. Black Letter Symptoms (Tyler-16)

- *RECTUM*—feels full; dryness and itching.
- Rectum feels full of small sticks (characteristic). (Coll.).
- Hard stool passed with difficulty, with dryness of rectum and heat. Stool followed by rectal fullness.
- Haemorrhoids—blind and painful, rarely bleeding.
- Haemorrhoids painful, burning, purplish, generally "blind".
- Pain in haemorrhoids like a knife, sawing up and down: could not sit, stand or lie, only kneel.

- "Some carry the nuts in their breeches' pockets as a preventive."
- *LEUCORRHOEA* with lameness in back across sacroiliac articulations, with great fatigue walking; that part of the back gives out when walking even a little way.
- "CHEST—Complaints of horses".
- Constant dull *BACKACHE*; walking almost impossible; scarcely able to stoop, or to rise after sitting.
- Constant headache affecting the sacrum and hips, much worse by walking or stooping forwards.
- Paralytic feeling in arms, legs and spine.
- Heaviness and lameness.
- Fullness in various parts.
- Mucous membranes dry and swollen; burn and feel raw.
- Glandular swellings of bone.

ATHUSA CYNAPIUM

I. Introduction (Cow-22)

Synonym: Aethusa Cynapium.
Natural Order: Umbelliferæ.
Common Names: Fools parley, Garden Hemlock.
Habitat: Common weed growing throughout Europe.
Preparation: Tincture from fresh plant when in flower.
Proved by Nenning, a Hahnemannian prover, in 1828.

II. General Analysis (Cow)

Classed as powerful narcotic poison now being claimed harmless. May provoke nausea, vomiting and other symptoms of gastro-intestinal irritation.

III. Suited to (Allen-21)

Especially children during dentition, in hot summer weather, children who can not bear milk. Great weakness of children/ cannot stand, unable to hold up head (Abrot.), prostration with sleepiness, expression of great anxiety and pain. Idiocy in children, incapacity to think.

IV. Clinical (Clarke-I-35)

Brain-fag, Cholera infantum, Convulsions, Cough, Delirium, Diarrhoea, Dyspepsia, Ear-discharge from, Epilepsy, Excoriations, Eye affections, Glands-affections of, Headache, Herpes, Hiccough, Idiocy, Infantile paralysis, Mind-weakness of, Sleeplessness, Stomach disordered, Trismus, Vomiting.

V. Symptoms-Particular (Nash-436)

1. One of the best remedies for vomiting in children.
2. Milk comes out as soon as it is swallowed, by great effort, after which child becomes relaxed and drowsy.

If milk remains down longer, it finally comes up in very sour curds, so large that it seems impossible that the child could have thrown them. If not checked, this condition develops into Cholera infantum, with green, watery or slimy stools, Colic and Convulsion (compare with large curd in Calc. c.). Convulsion are peculiar-eyes turn downwards, not upwards or sideways.

3. If the case goes on unfavourably then there is an appearance of sunkenness in the face with linea nasalis, which is a surface of pearly whiteness on upper lips, bounded by a distinct line from the outer nasal orifice to the angles of the mouth. This is a key symptom.
4. *Complete absence of thirst.* Prostration and anxiety well marked, but absence of thirst rules out Ars.
5. Imagines a rat or mouse run across the room. (Symptom found in hard worked, nervous women).

VII. Black Letter Symptoms (Tyler-19)

- Drawn condition, beginning at the ala nasi, and extending to the angle of the mouth, gives the face an expression of great anxiety and pain.
- Intolerance of milk: the children throw up their milk almost as soon as swallowed, curdled or not curdled, in ten to fifteen minutes, by a sudden and violent vomiting; then weakness makes them drowsy for some minutes
- Vomiting curdled milk.

AGARICUS MUSCARIUS

I. Introduction (Cow-23)

Synonym: Amanita
Natural Order: Fungi.
Common Names: Bug Agaric, Fly Agaric.
Habitat: Poisonous mushroom growing in dry pine and birch forests of Europe, Asia and America.
Preparation: Tincture from entire younger fresh plant.

II. General Analysis (Cow)

Acts upon circulation, respiration, peristalsis (characteristic movement of intestine) and secretion. Paralysis results from large doses. Anaemia of nerve centres caused by persistent spasm of blood vessels. Effects on motor sensory centres cause tremor, Chorea (jerky movements), convulsion. Effects from sensory pain in spinal cord and nerve, tenderness of/to touch especially in lumber region/spine.

III. Suited to (Allen-22)

Persons with light hair, lax muscles, old people, drunkards with their headaches. Headache. Bad affects after a debauch (Lobel., Nux. v., Ran. b.)

IV. Clinical (Clarke-I-39)

Acne rosacea, Blepharospasm, Brain softening, Bunions, Chilblains, Chorea, Coldness, Cough, Cramps, Delirium tremens, Dysmenorrhoea, Enteric fever, Epilepsy (with great exertion of strength), Fistula lachrymalis, Gangrene, General paralysis, Hyperpyrexia, Itching, Jaundice, Lichen, Lumbago, Meningitis, Myopia, Neuralgia, Numbness, Nystagmus, Phthisis, Rheumatism, Sacrum-pain in, Sebaceous tumours, Sexual excess-effects of, Spinal Irritation, Spleen-affections of, Starting, Stitch in side, Tic convulsif, Toothache, Tremors, Typhoid fever, Typhus.

V. Symptoms-General (Nash-459)

1. Ears, face, nose and skin in general, red and itch as if from chilblains.
2. Twitching in eyelids (especially), face, extremities; even choreaic jerking, which cease during sleep.
3. Spinal column painful, sensitive to touch, aching extending to lower limbs.

VI. Symptoms-Particular (Nash-459)

1. Ear, face, nose, toes and skin with redness, itching and burning as if from being frozen.
2. Twitching in eyelids, face, to severe twitching / cases of chorea.

VII. Black Letter Symptoms (Tyler 24-25)

- Delirium Tremens.
- Delirium with constant raving.
- Dull, drawing HEADACHE in morning, extending in to root, with nosebleed or thick mucous discharge.
- Headaches of those who are subject to Chorea; or who readily become delirious in fever or with pain; twitching or grimaces.
- Redness, burning itching of EARS, as if they had been frozen.
- TONGUE dry.
- Very drowsy after dinner, quite unusual; he SLEEPS very deeply and gets awake with pains in all limbs.
- Sudden convulsive COUGHS, < forenoons, or during day.
- Pain in LUMBAR REGION AND SACRUM: and while sitting; pain, sore aching, back not sensitive to touch.
- Burning itching on both HANDS, as if frozen; parts hot, swollen, red.
- Trembling of hands.
- Stiffness in fingers from gout.
- Twitching of gluteal muscles.
- Pain in bones of lower LEGS. Sometimes as if in the periosteum.

- Pain and inflammation of frost-bitten toes.
- Chilblains.
- Tearing in limbs < in rest or sitting, > moving.
- Pains in limbs with lameness and numbness.
- Uncertainty in walking, tumbling over everything in the way.
- Twitching of eyelids and eyeballs; of cheeks; in chest posteriorly; in abdomen.
- Involuntary movements (especially with children) while awake; Ceasing during sleep.
- Spasmodic motions, from simple involuntary motions and jerks of single muscles, to a dancing of whole body, Chorea.
- Paralysis of upper and lower limbs, incipient softening of spinal marrow.
- During sleep, one does not notice any motion of eyes whatever in clonic spasms of eyes.
- Chilblains, Frost-bite, all consequences of exposure to cold. esp. in face.
- Shiverings over body, run from above downward.
- Shudders; with bitter vomiting after supper.
- Sweat on walking, on slightest exertion.
- Profuse sweat.
- Burning, itching, redness and swelling, as from Frost-bite.
- Drunkards, especially for their headaches.

ALLIUM CEPA

I. Introduction (Cow-32)

Natural Order: Liliaceae.
Common Name: Onion
Habitat: Universal garden vegetable.
Preparation: Tincture from fresh common red onion.

It was first proved in 1847 by Dr. Herring and provings were published ten years later (Pierce-233).

II. General Analysis (Cow)

Acts esp. upon conjunctiva, and the respiratory mucous membrane, producing highly irritated condition resembling an acute catarrh. It also produces Catarrhal conditions of the intestinal tract.

III. Suited to (Allen-24)

Acute catarrhal inflammation of mucous membranes, with increased secretion. Catarrhal dull headache with coryza < evening, > open air, < on returning to a warm room (Sul., Puls.) person with coryza profuse watery and acrid nasal discharge with profuse watery bland discharge from eyes.

IV. Clinical (Clarke-I-53)

Anus-fissure of, Ascites, Catarrh, Colds, Coryza, Cough, Diarrhoea, Facial paralysis, Feet-easily galled, Hay-fever, Hernia, Influenza, Laryngitis, Panaritium, Pneumonia, Trauma, Whitlow, Whooping-cough, Yellow fever.

V. Symptoms-General (Nash-443)

1. Cold extends to the bronchi, with profuse secretion of mucus; coughing and much rattling (Chel.).

2. Coryza with frequent sneezing and profuse acrid discharge, corroding upper lip and nose, Lachrymation also profuse but bland. (Euph. reverse).
3. Modalities: < in the evening and in warm room, > in open air (the coryza).

VI. Symptoms-Particular (Nash-444)

1. Onion cut affect on eyes and nose, profuse lachrymation with burning, biting and smarting of the eyes, but bland discharge (does not sore eyes afterwards). Euph.-acrid discharge from eye, bland from nose.
2. Cold-Frequent and constant sneezing, with profuse acrid discharge, which burns and corrodes, the nose and upper lip, and it is worse in evening and indoors and better in open air.

ALOE SOCCOTRINA

I. Introduction (Cow-34)

Synonym: Aloe Socotrina.
Natural Order: Liliaceae.
Habitat: a succulent plant of Africa.
Preparation: Tincture from inspissated juice.

II. General Analysis (Cow)

Acts upon liver, muscular portion of large intestine, rectum (causing intense congestion). Chief action-upon rectum.

III. Suited to (Allen-25)

Indolent, weary persons, averse to either mental or physical labour. Mental labour fatigues. Old people, esp. Old women of relaxed phlegmatic habit. Extreme prostration with perspiration.

IV. Clinical (Clarke-I-60)

Abdomen-plethora of, Anus-affections of, Bronchitis, Colic, Constipation, Cough, Diarrhoea, Dysentery, Gleet, Gonorrhoea, Haemorrhoids, Hysteria, Lumbago, Onanism-effects of, Phthisis, Proctitis, Prolapsus uteri, Prostate-affections of, Sacrum-pain in, Tenesmus.

V. Symptoms-General (Nash-319)

1. Insecurity of rectum; rectum feels full of heavy fluid, which will fall out, and does, if he does not go to stool immediately. Diarrhoea.
2. Solid stool, passing (in large balls) away involuntarily and unnoticed.
3. Great fullness and weight in whole abdomen, with feeling of weight in rectum and haemorrhoids

protruding like a bunch of grapes > by cold water applied.

VI. **Symptoms-Particular** (Nash-319)

Aloe. = Podo.-as cathartics.
—Diarrhoea during hot weather < in the morning, well supplemented by Sul.

Aloe. Stool

1. Yellow, faecal, bloody with transparent jelly like mucous (Kali bich.) sometimes in great mass or gobs, drops out of rectum almost unnoticed.
2. Stool with flatus or urine, involuntarily.
3. The rectum full of heavy fluid which escapes if not attended to at once.
   Olean.,
   Mur. a.
4. Rectum protrudes like bunch of grapes > cold water (Mur. a. > hot water).
5. Great rumbling in abdomen before stool and heaviness in rectum is sometimes felt in whole pelvis and abdomen as well.
6. < Walking, eating, drinking with clammy sweat, heat in rectum, weakness.
7. Blue Haemorrhoids —itch intensely-Aloe.
   —very sore and sensitive to touch-Mur. a.
8. Stool unnoticed in diarrhoea (even in constipation).
9. Alternate Diarrhoea and Constipation
   Ant. c.,
   Aloe.

ALUMINA

I. Introduction (Cow-37)

Synonym: Aluminium tri-hydrate
Common Name: Pure clay.
Preparation: Triturations

II. General Analysis (Cow)

Affects directly the motor-nervous system giving rise to a paralytic condition. Its most specific action is upon mucous membranes esp. of intestine and vagina. The condition seems to be that of extreme dryness and lack of secretion, with more or less irritation.

III. Suited to (Allen-27)

Persons who suffer from chronic diseases. Constitutions deficient in animal heat (Calc. c., Sil.) spare, dry, thin, dark complexioned, with cheerful disposition, hypochondria, dry, tettery, itching of whole body when getting warm in bed (Sul.). Itching worse in winter. "Acon. of the chronic diseases".

IV. Clinical (Clarke-I-67-68)

Anus-affections of, Boils, Bubo, Catarrh, Chlorosis, Constipation, Constipation-of suckling, Cough, Disappointments-effects of, Dysentery, Dyspepsia, Eczema, Eyes-affections of, Fissures, Fistula, Headache, Hernia, Irritation, Leucorrhoea, Locomotor ataxy, Nails-affections of, Otorrhoea, Ozaena, Paralysis, Pregnancy-constipation of; toothache of, Prostatorrhoea, Rhagades, Scrofula, Strabismus, Taste disordered, Tetters-moist and itching, Throat-affections of, Trismus, Typhus.

V. **Symptoms-General** (Nash-379)

1. Inactivity of the rectum; even the soft stool requires great straining.
2. Anaemia in women who are hungry for starch, chalk rags, charcoal, cloves and other ridiculous unnatural things; potatoes disagree; profuse leucorrhoea
3. Great heaviness in lower limbs, weak, has to sit down; numbness of heels; sense of hot iron thrust through back.

VI. **Symptoms-Particular** (Nash-379)

1. Inactivity of rectum-Soft stool needs straining.
   Sep. (Allen-28)
   Bry.-no desire due to dryness of mucous follicles, of dry, spare subjects; lack of expulsive power (Anac., Sep., Sil., Verat.)
2. Exhausted after Menses. Menses scanty, delayed, pale coloured, and she is exhausted and pale after them. Patient is weak, must sit down to rest.
   Alumina, Carb. a., Cocc.
3. As Profuse as Menses-Leucorrhoea-running down to heel
   Day-Alumina
   Night-Syph. (Allen-28)
4. Infantile constipation-(of bottle fed babies), of old people—
   Lyc.
   Op. (Allen-28)
5. Haemorrhage from bowels-in Typhoid fever-blood in large solid clots.
6. Craves Unusual-Alum-chalk etc. No potato
   —Nat. m.-No bread
   —Puls.-No FAT.
7. Sensation of constriction in throat and also phlegm hurts to swallow.
   Sore throat-Clergyman's sore throat, raw, better hot drink and food.
   Arg. n.,

Hep. s.,
Dolichos.,
Nit. ac.
Phyt. (All have splinter-like in throat sensation.)

8. Dryness in throat causes continual disposition to hack, and after long time patient raises a little and tough mucous.
9. Heaviness of lower limbs—drags them while walking, staggers, even has to sit down.
10. Numbness of the heel when stepping, can walk only with eyes open and day time.

VII. Black Letter Symptoms (Tyler-36)

- Eyes-inflamed; itching at inner canthus; agglutination at night, lachrymation by day. Burning; dryness; smarting
- Yellow halo round the candle.
- Eyelids-thickened, dry, burning.
- Redness of nose.
- Point of nose cracked.
- Involuntary spasmodic twitching of lower jaw; with haemorrhage of bowels, and dark offensive stools.
- In evening, dryness of throat, which induces frequent clearing of throat.
- Worse from eating Potatoes.
- Painter's colic.
- Inactivity of rectum; even the soft stool needs great straining
- Rectum seems paralysed.
- No desire for, and no ability to, pass stool till there is a large accumulation.
- Stools; hard, knotty, covered with mucus; like sheep's dung, with cutting in anus, followed by blood ; like pipe-stems.
- Soft and thin stool, passing with difficulty.
- Severe haemorrhage from bowels, with flow of urine.
- Diarrhoea whenever she urinates.
- Evacuation of a small quantity of hard faeces, with pressure and a sensation of excoriation in the rectum.

- Urine voided when straining at stool; or cannot pass urine without straining.
- Constipation of sucklings.
- Continual, dry, hacking cough, with vomiting and arrest of breathing; with frequent sneezing.
- Every morning a long attack of dry cough, ends with difficult raising of a little white mucus.
- Great heaviness in lower limbs; he can scarcely drag them.
- When walking he staggers and has to sit down.
- Great wariness of the legs when sitting.
- Faint and tired; must sit down.

AMMONIUM CARBONICUM

I. Introduction (Cow-43)

Synonym: Sesqui = carbonate of Ammonia.
Common Name: Smelling salt, Salvolatile.
Preparation: Solution in water.
Hahnemann used this medicine in 30th potency.

II. General Analysis (Cow.)

Has profound influence upon the blood, producing liquefaction giving rise to Haemorrhage and great prostration. Through ganglionic nervous system, without affecting the brain, produces increased activity of the heart, arteries and to some extent nearly all organs of the body. Chief action-intense congestion and inflammation of gastro-intestinal and respiratory mucous lining.

III. Suited to (Allen-30)

Haemorrhagic diathesis, stout fleshy women leading sedentary life; delicate women, who must have smelling bottle at hand, readily catch cold in winter. Children dislike washing (Ant. c., Sul.) Loses breath when falling asleep; must awaken to get breath (Grind., Lach.).

IV. Clinical (Clarke-I-84)

Asthma, Bronchitis, Cough, Dislocations-pains from, Emphysema, Enuresis, Erysipelas, Gums-sensitive, Haemorrhoids, Hysteria, Lungs-oedema of, Measles, Miliary eruption, Nose affections, Parotitis, Rickets, Scarlatina, Spotted fever, Sprain, Sternum-pain on, Toothache, Uraemia, Whitlow.

V. Symptoms-General (Nash-433)

1. Nose-bleed when washing the face in the morning.

2. Tendency to gangrenous degeneration of glands, as in Scarlatina; the parotids.
3. Weak, anaemic, flabby women. Weak, no reaction, addicted to the smelling bottle.

VI. Symptoms-Particular (Nash-433)

1. Dry stuffed coryza, < Night, has to breathe through mouth;
   Amm. c.,
   Samb.,
   Lyc.,
   Nux. v.,
   Stict.
2. Epistaxis-while washing face:
   Amm. c.,
   Kali c.
3. Scarlatina-(throat seems to be the centre) body red, almost bluish red.
   Amm. c.,
   Zinc.-Convulsion with above symptoms.
4. Erysipelas of old people, cerebral symptoms simulating a drunken stupor.

VII. Black Letter Symptoms (Tyler-43)

- Sense of oppressive fullness as if the forehead could burst.
- Nose bleed from left nostril. When washing hands or face in a.m.
- Nose-stoppage at night mostly, must breathe though mouth.
- Rabid HUNGER, yet satiated after having eaten a little. A good deal of hunger and appetite.
- Heat in face after and during dinner.
- Qualmishness.
- One of the best remedies in Emphysema.
- Cough at night-every morning at 3 AM; dry from tickling of throat, as of dust.
- Angina pectoris.
- Right ARM-appeared to weigh a hundred weight and without strength.

- Spasm in right arm which drew it backwards.
- Panaritium; finger inflamed. Deep seated pariosteal pain.
- Better for external pressure; headache better, constrictive pain in the stomach better, pain in bowels better.
- Body-red, as if covered with Scarlatina.
- Scarlatina-malignant with somnolence etc.
- Body feels bruised.

AMMONIUM MURIATICUM

I. Introduction (Cow-48)

Synonym: Ammonium chloride.
Common Name: Sal Amoniac.
Preparation: Solution-also Trituration.

II. General Analysis (Cow)

Acts upon blood and promotes glandular secretion. Increases the elimination of urea. Chief action-upon mucous membranes whose secretions are greatly increased.

III. Suited to (Allen-32)

Fat and sluggish persons, or body large and fat, but legs too thin. Hamstrings feel painfully short when walking, tension in joints as if from shortening of muscles (Caust., Cimex.).

IV. Clinical (Clarke-I-91)

Anosmia, Bronchitis, Constipation, Coryza, Cough, Diarrhoea, Eyes inflamed, Feet-pain in, Glands enlarged, Haemorrhoids, Liver-affections of, Melancholia, Menstruation disordered, Pneumonia, Sciatica, Scurvy, Spleen-pain in, Sprain, Stumps-neuralgia in, Tonsils-swelling of, Ulcers.

V. Symptoms-Particular (Nash-435)

1. Sensation of coldness in back and between shoulders-(Generally found in chest affections such as cough or pain in chest without cough.)
   Amm. mur.,
   Phos., }
   Lyc. } burning between shoulders.

2. Constipation-stools dry, hard, crumbling, coated with mucous, [excellent remedy (Cow.-50)] very difficult to expel.
   Amm. c. -loose stool
   Caust. -covered with mucous, as if greased.
3. Sensation and pain as if muscles were contracted:
   Amm. mur.,
   Caust.-actual arthritis deformans, (Nat. m., Cimex.-arthritis deformans)
4. Menses of blood from uterus at Night:
   Amm. mur.,
   Bov.
5. Menses flows on when:
   Kreos. -lying down, ceases when sitting or walking.
   Lil. t. -moving about, ceases when she stops.
   Mag. c.-in night or lying, ceases when walking.
6. Pain in heels-as if ulcerated:
   Amm. c.,
   Phyt.,
   Cycl.,
   Mang.,
   Caust.,
   Led.,
   Valer.
7. Sciatica- < when sitting. Some feel better when walking,
   > entirely relieved when lying.

AMYLENUM NITROSUM

I. Introduction (Cow-51)

Synonym: Nitrite of Amyl.
Preparation: Dilutations made with alcohol.

II. General Analysis (Cow)

Acts powerfully upon motor centres of the spinal cord, allowing a passive congestion of cerebral vessels, respiratory and circulatory organs. Respiration becomes deep, laboured, rapid, and action of heart extremely violent. Chief characteristic-Headache, throbbing and fullness sensation. Heart-aching pain, constriction.

III. Suited to (Allen-32)

Nervous, plethoric women after menopause-Craving fresh air, flushing. Craves for fresh air; even in coldest weather opens windows (Arg. n., Lach., Sul.), opens clothing, removes bed coverings. Flushing starts from face to various parts of body, often followed by profuse, hot sweats. Parts below cold. Great prostration after. Face flushed after slight emotion(Coca, Ferr.). Blushing-Chronic/acute/sea sickness. Collar seems too tight (Lach.). Profound and repeated yawning (Kali c.). Tumultuous heart action-intense throbbing (Glon.). Constant stretching for hours, impossible to satisfy the desire.

IV. Clinical (Clarke-I-98)

Angina pectoris, Blushing, Chorea, Climacteric flushing, Epilepsy, Exophthalmos, Flushing, Headache, Heart affections, Hysteria, Sea-sickness, Sunstroke.

V. Symptoms-Particular (Nash-455)

1. Arrests paroxysms of epilepsy.
2. Resuscitating patients sinking under anaesthesia.
3. Chronic blushing on least excitement.
4. Tumultuous heart action (Similar Glon.).

ANACARDIUM ORINTALE

I. Introduction (Cow-53)

Synonym: Anacardium Orientale.
Natural Order: Anacardeiceae.
Common Name: Marking Nut.
Habitat: A small tree in East Indies.
Preparation: Tincture from crushed seed.

This drug was proved by Hahnemann who said that "during last one thousand years" this medicine "had fallen in total oblivion" (Chronic Diseases I-p-277)

II. General Analysis (Cow.)

Acts directly upon sensorium, depressing the cerebral centres, producing general nervous prostration. Chief characteristics:

1. Loss of memory (near exam esp.)
2. Sensation of plug in different parts.

III. Suited to (Allen-34)

Person with lack of confidence in himself and others. Feels as if he had two wills-pulling in opposite directions. When walking he is conscious that some one is following him, suspects everything around him. Sudden loss of memory, Everything seems to be in dream. He is greatly troubled about his forgetfulness. Irresistible desire to curse and swear (Lac. can., Lil. t., Nit. ac., stram—wants to pray continually). Strange temper, laughs in serious matters and serious in laughable matters. Sudden loss of memory.

IV. Clinical (Clarke-I-101)

Alcoholism, Apoplexy, Brain-fag, Constipation, Cough, Debility, Dysmenorrhoea, Dyspepsia, Eczema, Elephantia-sis, Examination funk, Haemorrhoids, Headache, Heart affections, Hypochondriasis, Hysteria, Insanity, Memory lost, Mind-weakness of, Nervous ailments, Palpitation, Paralysis, Pemphigus, Rheumatism, Self-abuse, Skin-diseases of, Smell-illusions of, Spinal affections, Stiff-neck, Vomiting of pregnancy, Whooping-cough, Warts, Writer's cramp.

V. **Symptoms-General** (Nash-375)

1. Pain in stomach when it is empty, relieved by eating.
2. Frequent ineffectual desire for stool, from insufficiency or paralytic state of rectum; with sense of lump or plug in anus; with the effort the desire vanishes.
3. Loss of memory; irresistible desire to curse and swear; feels as if he had two wills, one commanding, the other forbidding, to do things.
4. Pain and sensation as of a blunt plug in different parts.
5. Suspects every one and everything around him; when walking he felt anxious, as if some one were pursuing him; weakness of all the senses.

VI. **Symptoms-Particular** (Nash-375)

1. Plug sensation in various parts.
2. Dyspepsia-Anac. > after eating
   -Nux. v.-when digestive process is over (This time is < for Anac.)
3. Stomach ache > eating soon after, better or relieved.
4. Constipation-Nux. v.-has desire but irregular action.
   -Anac.-desire but insufficient action to carry out; with action desire goes.
5. Loss of memory (esp.) in old people of broken down constitutions.
   -Anac.-curses or swears.
   -Stram.-Prays continually.
6. Similar sensations
   -Anac.-of plug and of hoop in inner parts.
   -Aesc. hip.-as of fullness.
   -Cact.-of constriction.

7. Two wills each pulling to different directions:
   - -Anac.,
   - -Plat.

VII. Black Letter Symptoms (Tyler-48)

- Great weakness of Memory.
- Loss of memory.
- Irresistible desire to curse and swear.
- Hypochondriasis.
- When walking he feels anxious, as if some one were pursuing him; he suspected everything around him.
- He is separated from the whole world; has no confidence in himself; despairs of being able to do that which is required of him.
- Weakness of all the senses.
- Pain Head, relieved entirely when eating: worse during motion and work.
- Gastric and nervous headaches.
- Dull pressure as from a plug, in left vertex upper border right orbit.
- Flat, offensive taste in Mouth.
- Symptoms disappear during dinner, but begin anew after two hours.
- Pain about Navel as if a blunt plug were squeezed into intestines.
- Great and urgent desire for stool, passed without evacuation.
- Rectum powerless, with sensation as if plugged up.
- Dull pressure as from a plug in right side chest.
- Cramp in calves when walking.
- Sensation as of a hoop or band round the part.
- Vision distinct.

ANTIMONIUM CRUDUM

I. Introduction (Cow-56)

Synonym: Ter-Sulphuret of Antimony.
Preparation: Trituration from crude Antimony after it has been pulverised under water.

It was first proved by Caspare, one of Hahnemann's provers (Pierce-249).

II. General Analysis (Cow.)

Acts powerfully upon all the mucous membranes and upon skin; most intensely upon intestinal mucous lining. chief characteristics are—milky white tongue, over loading of stomach, fretful, peevish disposition, does not want to be touched, alternate diarrhoea, esp. of old people, Headache after river bath, sore cracked nostrils and corners of mouth.

III. Suited to (Allen-37)

Children, young people inclined to grow fat (Calc. c.); for extremes of life. Old people with morning diarrhoea suddenly become constipated or alternate diarrhoèa and constipation. Sadness with weeping. Sensitive to cold, after taking cold bath, headache after river bathing.

IV. Clinical (Clarke-I-121)

Anus-irritation of, Callosities, Catarrh, Chorea, Constipation, Corns, Diarrhoea, Dyspepsia, Eczema, Feet-sore and horny, Fever, Gum-rash, Nails-degeneration of, Nettlerash, Piles, Prolapsus recti, Red-gum, Remittent fever, Stomach disordered, Sunstroke, Tendons inflamed, Tongue coated, Voice-low, Warts, Whooping-cough.

V. **Symptoms-General** (Nash-35)

1. Thick, milky white coating on tongue (in many complaints).
2. Derangement from over loading the stomach, especially fat food; nausea.
3. Crushed finger nails; grow in splits like warts and with horny spots.
4. Corns and callosities on soles, with excessive tenderness, can only walk with pain and suffering.
5. Alternate constipation and diarrhoea in old people, especially with the characteristic tongue.
6. Child cannot bear to be touched or looked at, fretful, cross.
7. Feverish conditions at night.
8. Headache; after river bathing; from taking cold, alcoholic drink. Deranged digestion; acids, fat, fruit. Suppressed Eruptions, mucous from anus, ichorous, oozing, staining yellow; mucous piles, cannot bear heat of sun; < from exertion in sun; exhausted in warm weather.

VI. **Symptoms-Particular** (Nash-36-39)

1. *Thickl* Towards Understanding Homeopathyy *coated white tongue.* A great stomach remedy disorders from over eating, with nausea, distress, Eructation taste of food eaten, he must "throw up for relief", a few globs of Ant. c. will often settle the business of suffering.
2. *Summer Diarrhoea* (stools partly solid and partly fluid)

   Bry. -< in morning on beginning to move.

   Ant. c.-alternate with constipation.
3. *Mucous piles*, continuous oozing of mucous staining the linen.
4. *Mental symptoms*:

   Child can't bear to be touched (Cham.-Reverse-wants to be carried).
5. High fever at Night with great thirst.
6. Sore, crusty nostrils, corners of the mouth.

7. *Finger nails grow in splits*-warts-with horny spots
   Sil.-nails crippled.
   Graph.-nails thick, crippled.
   Thuj. -Brittle (don't repair, go out of shape) Crumbling, distorted.
   Ant. c.-corns and callosities on soles can not walk. VERY TENDER
   Toe nails-brittle, grow out of shape, shrivel up, don't grow at all.
8. *Excessive Tenderness of Soles of the feet*:
   Ant. c. -Corns or callosities on sole.
   Baryt. c. -Sweat foot cause sore-soles.
   Puls. - pain and are tender.
   Led. - heels and soles tender when walking.
   Medo. - can walk on knees only
   Lyc. - Swollen and painful.
9. *Troubles by heat of sun*: exhausted during warm weather, cough worse when coming to warm room, gastric troubles, come on or are worse (Bry.) such as nausea, diarrhoea, vomiting. Cold bathing < troubles; child cries when washed in cold water, headache, gastric troubles worse. Beginning of Trouble from falling in water.
   Bry.,
   Glon.,
   Gels.,
   Nat. c.,
10. Cough < Summer < from open air to room < heat of sun.
    Bry.,
    Ant. c..
11. Cold bathing < trouble aggravates.
    Ant. c.-< river bathing < falling in river, beginning of trouble from.
    Rhus t.,
    Sul.
12. Bleeding from bowels with solid faeces.
13. Chronic Redness of Eyelids.
14. Toothache in decayed tooth < night.
15. Gastric < acids, sour wine etc.

16. Taste of food in eructation. Must throw up for relief.

VII. Black Letter Symptoms (Tyler-53-54)

- Peevish. Sulky. Loathing of life.
- Child fretful, peevish, turns away and cries when touched
- Headache: after bathing; from deranging stomach, alcoholic drinks, after a chill; suppressed Eruption; from a cold.
- Eyes-soreness of outer canthi. Redness and inflammation of eyelids. Chronic blepharophthalmia of children.
- Sore, cracked and crusty *Nostrils*.
- Suppurating and long lasting eruption on Cheeks.
- Toothache, in hollow *Teeth*: Pain sometimes penetrates into head. Worse at night, after eating and from cold water: touching tooth with tongue causes pain as if nerve torn; better walking in open air.
- Gnawing pain in carious teeth; after every meal.
- TONGUE coated; thick white; milky white, yellow.
- White tongue.
- Lips dry. Cracks in the corners of mouth, painful like sores.
- Gums detach from teeth and bleed easily.
- STOMACH: Violent thirst, with dryness of lips.
- Thirst in the evening with desire to drink.
- Gulping up of food, tasting of the ingesta.
- Stomach weak. Easily disturbed digestion.
- Gastric catarrh: white tongue; nausea and vomiting.
- Very liquid STOOLS.
- Diarrhoea: watery with undigested food: watery with little hard lumps, Worse from vinegar, acids, sour wine; overheating; after cold bathing; at night and early morning.
- Diarrhoea of old people.
- Alternate diarrhoea and constipation of old people.
- Difficult, hard stool; faeces too large.
- Elderly people with diarrhoea, all at once get costive.

- Mucous piles, pricking, burning; continuous mucous discharge, staining yellow. Sometimes ichor oozes out.
- COUGH: first attack is always most severe, subsequent ones weaker and weaker; (whooping cough).
- Pain in chest with heat.
- Blenorrhoea pulmonum, or phthisis mucosa.
- Severe continual itching on chest the whole day.
- Violent itching on BACK.
- Arthritic pain in FINGERS.
- Drawing pains in fingers and their joints.
- Drawing pain in the left hip-joints.
- Large horny places on soles, close to toes.
- Great sensitiveness of soles when walking.
- Great SLEEPINESS during the day, mostly forenoon.
- Exhausted in warm weather.
- Cannot bear HEAT of sun.
- Worse overheating near the fire.
- After overheating, diarrhoea.
- Sensitive to COLD: to inhaling cold air; after taking cold.
- Pertussis, worse cold washing.
- Cold bathing: causes violent headache: cold in head; gastric catarrh; diarrhoea; suppressed menses
- Violent chill without thirst; heat with thirst followed by sweat.
- After the sweat is over, heat and thirst return.
- Belching with taste of what has been eaten.
- Constant discharge of wind, up and down, immediately reproduced for years (cured case).
- FEVER; heat attended by sweat.
- Gastric Fever.
- Gastric symptoms predominate: disgust for drink and food, bitter mouth and vomit.
- Loathing, nausea and desire to vomit.
- Vomiting.
- Vomiting after sour wine.
- After vinegar or acid wine, loose stools.
- Mucous membranes generally affected.
- Measles-like Eruption: or measles delayed: vomiting during measles.
- Horny excrescences.

ANTIMONIUM TARTARICUM

I. Introduction (Cow-60)

Synonym: Tartarate of Antimony and Potash.
Common name: Tartar Emetic.
Preparation: Alcoholic dilution from a watery solution or trituration from a pure crude tartar emetic.
Some of its symptoms were proved by Hahnemann (Pierce-252)

II. General Analysis (Cow.)

Acts directly upon nerve centre at the base of the brain; respiratory system, mucous membranes of stomach, liver and lungs. On mucous membranes-catarrhal inflammations or pustular inflammation. Chief characteristics are (Pierce-Plain Talks) accumulation of rattling mucous in the chest with vomiting, Cold clammy sweat esp. on forehead, profound depression of heart, pulse, temperature, great sleepiness (Apis., Gels., Nux. m.) (Allen).

III. Suited to (Allen-39)

Torpid, phlegmatic persons with hydrogenoid constitution, Diseases originating from damp places (Ars., Aran., Tereb.).

IV. Clinical (Clarke-I-128)

Alcoholism, Aphthae, Asphyxia neonatorium, Asthma, Bilious affections, Bronchitis, Catarrh, Chicken-pox, Chol-era, Cholera morbus, Coccygodynia, Cough, Croup, Delirium tremens, Dyspepsia, Ecthyma, Eyes inflamed, Impetigo, Intermittent fever, Laryngitis, Lumbago, Lung affections, Myalgia, Paralysis agitans, Plica-polonica, Pneumonia, Psoriasis, Rheumatism, Ringworm, Screaming, Small-pox, Stiff-neck, Sycosis, Synovitis, Taste disordered,

Thirst, Tongue coated, Tremors, Varioloid, Vomiting, Whooping-cough.

V. Symptoms-General (Nash-235)

1. Great accumulation of mucous in the air passages with coarse rattling with inability to expectorate; impending paralysis of lungs.
2. Face very pale or cyanotic from unoxidized blood.
3. Great coma or sleepiness in most complaints.
4. Vomiting, intense nausea, with prostration; general coldness, cold sweat and sleepiness.
5. Trembling; internal head and hands.
6. Thick Eruption like pocks, often pustular; as large as a pea.
7. Modalities > from expectoration.
8. Both ends of life, childhood and old age; clings to those around; wants to be carried; cries and whines if any one touches him; will not let you feel the pulse.

VI. Symptoms-Particular (Nash-235)

1. A powerful emetic. (Nausea as strong as in Ipec. but not as persistent.)
2. Relief after vomiting.
   Ipec.-never relief, persistent nausea.
   Iris v.-ropy mucous (237) sour; Cholera Infantum.
3. Cholera Morbus—loose stool, cold, stupor, drowsiness, sweat.
   Ant. tar. -Specific.
   Cupr. -Cramp with above symptoms.
4. Great accumulation of mucous in respiratory organ with rattling, unable to raise it.
5. Great sleepiness (237) or drowsiness, sometimes amounting to coma.
   Op.,
   Nux. m.,
   Ant. tar.
6. Pneumonia with sleepiness.
   Op.-face darkened, sighing or slowed respiration.
   Nux. m.

7. Hepatization of the lungs after pneumonia:
   Ant. tar. (one of the best remedies) (Nash-237)
   Sul.-for absorption. If it fails then Ant. tar. (237)

VII. Black Letter Symptoms (Tyler-67-69)

- Bad Humour.
- The child wants to be carried (Cham.), cries if anyone touches it; will not let you feel the pulse.
- Dim, swimming eyes.
- Pallor. Pale, sunken face.
- Rheumatic toothache of intermitting type.
- During dentition, catarrhal hyperaemia.
- Tongue very red, dry in the middle.
- Tongue red in streaks.
- Tongue covered with thick, white, pasty coat.
- Much mucous in throat with short breathing.
- Disgust for food, frequent nausea and relief by vomiting.
- Belching which relieves.
- Nausea causes great anxiety.
- Continuous anxious nausea, straining to vomit, with sweat on the forehead.
- Nausea, vomiting and loss of appetite. Vomits with great effort.
- Absence of thirst.
- Absence of thirst the whole day.
- Vomiting, followed by great languor, drowsiness, loathing, and desire for cooling things.
- Great precordial anxiety with vomiting of mucus and bile.
- Sharp cutting colic before stool.
- Child at birth pale, breathless, gasping, though the cord still pulsates.
- The mucus rattles in the chest.
- Rattling of mucus when coughing or breathing.
- Rattling originates in upper bronchi and can be heard at a great distance.
- Much rattling of mucus in trachea; cannot get it up.
- Shortness of breath from suppressed expectoration, especially if drowsy.

- Unequal breath, now shorter, then longer, much more frequent when lying. Better when child is carried upright.
- Respiration with great rattling of mucus.
- Suffocated and oppressed about 3 AM, Must sit up to get air; better after cough and expectoration.
- Cough compels the patient to sit up, is moist and rattling, but without expectoration.
- When the child coughs there appears to be a large collection of mucus in the bronchial tubes, and it seems as if much would be expectorated, but nothing comes up.
- Coughing and gaping consecutively, particularly children, with crying or dozing, and twitching of the face.
- Profuse mucus with feeble expulsive power (Bronchitis in infants and old people).
- Profuse mucus sputa, easily expectorated.
- Cough grows less frequent, patient shows signs of "carbonised blood".
- Rattling of phlegm on chest, better when carried in an upright position, worse lying down; with oppression.
- Inflammation of respiratory mucus membrane.
- Sputa blood-streaked, rust coloured, adhering like glue to the vessel.
- Atalectasis, with symptoms of asphyxia belonging to the remedy; with oedema of unhepatized portions of the lungs; breathing laboured, orthopnoea, mucus rattles.
- Oedema of lungs. Emphysema. Impending paralysis of lungs.
- Grippe: acute pneumonia; broncho-pneumonia: pleuro-pneumonia.
- Pulse hard, full, strong; sometimes trembling; very much accelerated with every motion.
- Pulse rapid, weak, trembling.
- Great restlessness. Tosses with anxiety.
- Prostration and collapse.
- Violent pain in lumbo-sacral region; the slightest

effort to move causes retching and cold clammy sweat.

- Trembling of hands.
- Great sleepiness: irresistible inclination to sleep, with nearly all affections.
- Coma, or, great sleeplessness.
- Worse at night and sleepless.
- Warmth aggravates; even getting warm in bed.
- Skin covered with a running, sticky sweat.
- The tissues it affects.
- Collection of synovia in joints.
- Mucus membranes; catarrhal inflammations; conjunctivitis; gastritis, enteritis; laryngitis, trachiitis, bronchitis, extending even into the air-cells, cystitis.
- Pustular Eruption; on conjunctiva, face, mouth and fauces, oesophagus, stomach, jejunum, genitals.
- Variola: backache, headache and cough; crushing weight on chest before eruptive stage. Also when the eruption fails. Diarrhoea etc. also when eruption fails.
- Chest, anterior surface of upper arms, wrists, abdomen and inner side thigh covered with closely set, bright-red, small, conic, hard pustules, with an inflamed tetter-like base, itching intolerably.
- Pustular eruption leaves bluish-red marks on face, etc.
- Thick eruption like pox, often pustular, as large as a pea.

APIS MELLIFICA

I. Introduction (Cow-64)

Synonym: Apis Mellifica.
Natural Order: Insecta (Clarke)
Common Name: Poison of honeybee.
Preparation: (1) Shaking live bees in a bottle and digesting them together with the poison emitted in alcohol 5 times their weight; allowed to remain a week, filtered tincture is 1st potency. (2) A tincture from the pure virus (Apium virus). The latter one was employed by Dr. Hoering in provings.

Apis was first proved in 1852 by Dr. Frederick Humphries. (Pierce-256).

II. General Analysis (Cow.)

Acts predominantly on kidneys, producing an acute inflammation. It causes oedema both of the skin and mucous membranes. It produces urticaria like eruption. It effects serous membranes, causing inflammations like hydrocephelus etc. Its main characteristics are—Burning stinging pains; prostration, Dropsy, Thirstlessness with burning heat, scanty Urine (H. Farrington).

III. Suited to (Allen-41)

Strumous constitutions, glands enlarged, indurated, open cancer, women esp. widows, children and girls who, generally careful, become awkward and let things fall while handling them.

IV. Clinical (Clarke-I-138)

Abscess, Ankles-swelling of, Apoplexy, Asthma, Bladder affections, Carbuncles, Chancre, Constipation-of suckling, Diarrhoea, Diphtheria, Dissection wounds, Dropsy,

Ear-erysipelas of, Erysipelas, Erythema nodosum, Eyes-affections of; optic neuritis, Feet burning, Gangrene, Gout, Hands swollen, Heart affections, Heat-spots, Housemaid's knee, Hydrocephalus, Hydrothorax, Injuries, Intermittent fever, Irritation, Jealousy-effect of, Joint-synoviitis of, Kidney-Bright's discase of, Labia-inflammation of, Laryngitis, Lichen, Meningitis, Menstruation disordered, Nettlerash, Nose-redness of, Operation-effects of, Ovaries-pain in; inflammation of; tumours of, Panaritium, Pannus, Peritonitis, Phlebitis, Pleurisy, Prostatitis, Punctured wounds, Red-gum, Rheumatism, Scarlatina, Self-abuse, Suppressed eruptions-effects of, Sycosis, Syphilis, Throat sore, Tongue-oedema of; ulceration of, Trachea-irritation in, Tumours, Typhus, Urethritis, Urine abnormal, Vaccination, Veins-varicose, Variola, Wounds.

V. **Symptoms-General** (Nash-143)

1. Burning, stinging pain (like bee stings); eyelids; throat; panaritium or felon, haemorrhoids, ovaries (especially right one), breasts (mastitis), skin (erysipelas; urticaria, Carbuncles).
2. Great oedema; general or local (face, ears, eyelids, especially lower); throat (diphtheria); genitals (especially scrotum); skin (erysipelas and urticaria); everywhere; general anasarca, abdomen. These oedemas are accompanied with the characteristic pains, or no pain at all.
3. Stupor, with sharp, sudden, shrill cries in brain disease (crieencephalique).
4. Thirstlessness, especially in Dropsy and during heat of intermittents.
5. Skin alternately dry and perspiring.
6. Suffocative; feels as if every breath would be his last especially in dropsical conditions or hot stage of intermittents.
7. Modalities < after sleep, on touch (very sensitive), from heat and warm room; > cold room or air and cold applications.
8. Bad effects from suppressed or retrocedent exanthemata; measles, scarlatina, urticaria.

9. Involuntary diarrhoea, with sensation as if anus were wide open.

VI. Symptoms-Particular (Nash-144-147)

1. Pains-Burning, Stinging. Burning pain > cold, Ars >hot.
2. Great Oedema-General or local, stupor.
3. Thirstlessness-
4. Skin.
5. Alimentary canal-Involuntary Diarrhoea.
6. *PAINS-BURNING STINGING*-Leading characteristic

   Apis.-> cold applications.
   Agar.-itch like chilblains.
   Ars., Sul.-Burning > hot.
7. *VIOLENT DIPHTHERIA*

   Apis.,
   Kali. bich.,
   Rhus t.
   Bap.-Painless throat affections with not so rapid swelling.
8. *LOCAL OEDEMA*

   Apis.-Mouth, throat, eye-lids, face, around eyes, lower lids.
   Phos.-Whole face
   Kali c.-Upper lid, like bag of water.
9. *THIRSTLESSNESS* (Leading symptom)

   Apis. -No Thirst.
   Acet. ac.,
   Ars., } with thirst.
   Apocy.
10. *SENSITIVE TO TOUCH* (as if bruised)

    Apis.-as if bruised (abdomen, uterus, ovarian regions etc.)
    China-whole body even hair
    Hep. s.-Erysipelas.
11. *BRAIN TROUBLE*

    Apis.-Deep stupor-often piercing screams or restless sleep.
    Alternately dry and hot or perspiring. Sensation as if every breath will be last.

VII. Black Letter Symptoms (Tyler-76)

- Vertigo and headache.
- Eyelids-Swollen, red and oedematous.
- No THIRST with heat.
- Sensation of rawness in the anus, with diarrhoea.
- STOOLS occur with every motion of the body as if the anus were constantly open.
- Sensation in the TOES and FOOT as if too large, swollen and stiff.
- MOST EXTREME SLEEPINESS.
- Closed rooms are perfectly intolerable.
- HEADACHE in warm room.
- INDICATIONS-SWELLING, OEDEMA, RELIEF from COLD, WORSE from HEAT, BURNING and STINGING PAINS.

ARGENTUM METALLICUM

I. Introduction (Cow-76)

Synonym: Pure metallic Silver.
Preparation: Triturations.
It was proved by Hahnemann. (Pierce-269)

II. General Analysis (Cow.)

Acts prominently upon mucous membranes of the digestive, respiratory and genitourinary tracts, upon spinal nerves causing pains in various parts, and a tendency to spasmodic action of muscles, upon glandular organs and heart. Its main characteristics are—General weakness lying down, Cough from laughing and talking; Much rawness and soreness when coughing, Arthralgia and arthritic inflammation of joints. Rheumatic pains in limbs and back when sitting, better lying, bones, cartilages, ligaments, (articulatory elements) Pains increase gradually, disappear suddenly (Arg. n., Caust.), Hoarseness of singers, Pain in Testicles (RH Farrington-613).

III. Suited to (Allen-43)

Tall, Thin, irritable persons, abuse of mercury, onanism-effects of.

IV. Clinical (Clarke-I-157)

Blepharitis, Brain-fag, Caries, Chlorosis, Cough, Diabetes, Enuresis nocturna, Epilepsy, Epithelial tissue-affections of, Exostosis, Heart affections, Hip-joint disease, Hysterical joint, Joint affections, Laryngitis, Ovaries-affections of, Phthisis, Pollutions, Rheumatism, Uterus-cancer of; prolapse of, Voice-loss of.

V. Symptoms-Particular (Nash-186)

1. Great weakness in the chest (Stan.)
2. Cough Worse from speaking, singing, laughing, reading, loud (197)
3. Testes- painful, swollen, sensitive to touch (Rodo, Clem, Pul, Spon) (363)

ARGENTUM NITRICUM

I. Introduction (Cow-79)

Synonym: Nitrate of Silver.
Preparation: First three decimal dilutions are made with distilled water; subsequent with alcohol.

It was proved by Hahnemann but he recorded only 16 symptoms Allen's encyclopaedia records 821 symptoms (Pierce-270).

II. General Analysis (Cow.)

An irritant poison, causing violent inflammation and ulceration of the throat, stomach and mucous membranes, primarily of the eyes, mouth, throat, upper air passages, the bowels and urethra causing violent congestion, destructive inflammation and ulceration of these tracts. Effect on nervous system causes prostration. It attacks and destroys R.B.Cs. causing general malnutrition, echymosis. Produces violent titanic Convulsion followed by paralysis. Main characteristics are (Lippe.)—withered dried up person. Always hurried.

III. Suited to (Allen-45)

Acute or chronic diseases from unusual or long continued mental exertion. Time passes slowly. (Cann. ind.). Apprehensive when ready on church or opera, diarrhoea sets in (Gels.).

IV. Clinical (Clarke-I-161)

Acidity, Addison's disease, Anaemia, Chancre, Dyspepsia, Epilepsy, Eructations, Erysipelas, Eye affections, Flatulence, Gastric ulcer, Gonorrhoea, Hands swollen, Headache, Heartburn, Impetigo, Locomotor ataxy, Neuralgia, Ophthalmia neonatorum, Paralysis, Prostate enlarged, Scarlatina, Small-pox, Spinal irritation, Syphilis,

Taste disordered, Throat-affections of, Tongue ulcerated, Warts, Zona.

V. Symptoms-General (Nash-293)

1. Impulsive; time goes too slow; must walk fast.
2. Apprehension, on getting ready for church, opera, etc; has an attack of diarrhoea.
3. Vertigo, with buzzing in the ears, and weakness and trembling.
4. Canthi, as red as blood; swollen, standing out like a lump of red flesh.
5. Irresistible desire for sugar; gastric ailments, with violent loud belching.
6. Stool; green, mucous, like chopped spinach in flakes; turn green on remaining on diaper; expelled with much spluttering.
7. Profuse, sometimes purulent, discharges from mucous membranes, generally.
8. Dried-up, withered patients, made so by disease.
9. Craves fresh air.

VI. Symptoms-Particular (Nash-294-299)

1. Lassitude (Kali c.)-Time goes too slow.
2. Apprehensive—when ready to go to an appointment-diarrhoea.
   Arg. n.,
   Gels.
3. Always Hurried, Impulsive.
   Arg. n.,
   Lil. t.
4. Hemicrania—Feeling of expansion, as if head was very large, better when tied up tight.
   Arg. n.,
   Puls.,
   Apis.
5. Vertigo—when looking up high at rise building, with buzzing in the ears and trembling.
   Arg. n. (Recent case).
   Gels.

6. Cannot walk with eyes closed.
7. Eye—Profuse purulent discharge, swollen eye lids from collection of Pus the eye.
   Apis.,
   Rhus t.(296).
   Purulent ophthalmia (Purulent matter pouring out on opening of the eyes).
   Arg. n., }
   Graph., } oftener in Blepharitis
   Staph., }
   Merc. c.,
   Bor.
8. Irresistible desire for sugar.
9. Gastric—Loud belching, noisy.
   Arg. n.,
   Carb. v.,
   China,
   After every meal, belching difficult, finally air rushes out with great noise and force.
10. Obstinate Diarrhoea—Green chopped mucus, Stools turn green in diaper, Stool with much spluttering.
   Calc. phos. (compare Calc. Phos. with Arg. n.)
   Spluttering stool with noisy flatus.
11. Hydrocephaloid. Bone development.
12. Wants sweets, Smoked meat.
13. Red painful tip of tongue, Papilla erect.
14. Throat—Tough mucus causes to hawk and hoarseness.
15. Backpain better walking but worse when getting up.
   Sul.,
   Caust.,
   Arg. n.
16. Epilepsy or Convulsion (299).
   Cupr. -restless between attacks.
   Arg. n. -before attacks, restless.

VII. Black Letter Symptoms (Tyler-80)

- Vertigo, general debility of limbs and trembling.
- Headache relieved by binding something tightly round head.

- Grey spot and bodies in shape of serpents move before vision.
- The cantha are as red as blood, caruncula is swollen.
- Painful red tip to tongue.
- Throat—Rawness and soreness.
- Thick tenacious mucous in throat.
- Sensation as if a splinter were lodged in throat when swallowing.
- Uvula and fauces dark red.
- Violent belching.
- Desire to vomit, with sensation as if head were in a vice.
- A slight colic wakes him up from a slight slumber, has sixteen evacuations with greenish mucous, with a quantity of noisy flatus.
- Violent diarrhoea, like spinach flakes.
- Four eructations of green mucous, with retching, vomiting of mucous.
- Tremulous weakness. Trembling and tremulous sensation.

ARNICA MONTANA

I. Introduction (Cow.-85)

Synonym: Arnica Montana.
Natural Order: Compositae.
Common Name: Leopard's Bane.
Habitat: Perennial herb in mountainous districts of N. hemisphere.
Preparation: Tincture from the root, leaves, flowers, mixed.

It was proved by Hahnemann and his fellow observers. Total 638 symptoms are recorded in MMP. The best known effect of this medicine is its remedial action in mechanical injuries, Hahnemann says this property of Arnica was known 200 years before he proved Arnica (Pierce-275).

II. General Analysis (Cow.)

Main action is upon blood, producing general anaemia and a tendency to Haemorrhage. It produces conditions similar to those resulting from injuries, falls, blows, even to traumatic fever, septicaemia by purulent infection. Its main characteristics are—bruised, sore feeling; compound Fracture.

III. Suited to (Allen-47)

Nervous women, sanguine plethoric persons, lively expression with red face; To those who remain long impressed by even slightest mechanical injuries; For the bad effects resulting from mechanical injuries even if received years back; Heat of upper part of body, lower part cold.

IV. Clinical (Clarke-I-171)

Abscess, Apoplexy, Back pains, Baldness, Bedsores, Black-eye, Boils, Brain-affections of, Breath foetid, Bronchitis, Bruises, Carbuncles, Chest-affections of, Chorea, Corns,

Cramps, Diabetes, Diarrhoea, Dysentery, Ecchymosis, Excoriations, Exhaustion, Eye affections, Feet sore, Haematemesis, Haematuria, Headache, Heart affections, Impotence, Labour, Lumbago, Meningitis, Miscarriage, Mental alienation, Miscarriage, Nipple sore, Nose affections, Paralysis, Pelvic hoematoccle, Pleurodynia, Purpura, Pyaemia, Rheumatism, Splenalgia, Sprain, Stings, Suppuration, Taste disordered, Thirst, Traumatic fever, Tumours, Voice-affections of, Whooping-cough, Wounds, Yawning.

V. Symptoms-General (Nash-386)

1. Bruised, Sore feeling all over, bed feels too hard.
2. Head, or head and face hot; body and extremities cold.
3. Ecchymoses as from bruises.
4. Stupor; answers, then falls back into stupor (Fever).
5. Taste and Eructation and stool, like rotten eggs.
6. Recent and remote affections from injuries, especially contusions or blows.
7. Haemorrhage, the result of mechanical injuries.

VI. Symptoms-Particular (Nash-386-90)

1. Bruises as if over all body-sensation of—
   Arn.—everything on which lies seems hard.
   Pyr.—must change his position to get relief.
   Bap.—as if lying on a board (stool offensive).
   Phyt.—sore and stiff; body can hardly move without groaning
   (throat prominent)
   Rhus t.—Soreness in every muscle, goes away with motion.
   Rut.—Parts on lies painful (actual injury in periosteumorbone)
   Staph.—Sore and weak limbs.
   China—Sprain like pain in bones and joints.
2. Many small boils, one after the other.
3. Fear of those coming near, of being struek or touched.
4. Stupor with voluntary urine and stools.

5. Flatus smelling like rotten egg. (eructation also)
6. Septicaemia-prevents.
7. Child cries-before coughing.
8. Putrid smell from mouth.
9. Results of Trauma-both acute and chronic-such as concussion, fracture of skull, headaches of long standing, meningitis, eyes inflammation with retinal Haemorrhage, blows on stomach, newly filled teeth epistaxis, retinal bleading etc.

VII. Black Letter Symptoms (Tyler-89-91)

- Stupor, with involuntary discharge of faeces.
- Forgetful; what he reads quickly escapes his memory, even the word he is about to speak.
- Says there is nothing the matter with him.
- Delirium tremens.
- Hopelessness; indifference. (After concussion).
- Fears being struck by those coming towards him; fears even the possibility of being touched (in gout).
- Violent attacks of anguish. (Angina pectoris)
- Vertigo when shutting eyes.
- Pressive headache as if head was being distended from within outward; pain seems to arise from something soft in vertex, with drawing in vertex and occiput, and tearing towards temples.
- Mechanical injuries; especially with stupor from concussion; Fracture of skull, or even compression (apply externally).
- Meningitis after mechanical or traumatic injuries, such as Concussion, bruises, falling, concussion of brain, etc., when suspecting exudetion of blood, fibrin or pus. In such cases we find great sopor and partial paralysis of tongue, oculmotors, iris or limbs.
- Meningitis after lesion or concussion, provided there is no complete want of reaction.
- Apoplexia sanguinea.
- Head feels too large.
- Eye—Inflammation of eyes, with suggillations after mechanical injuries.

- Retinal haemorrhage; expedites absorption of clots.
- A variety of eye troubles resulting from blows and various injuries; some times applied locally (tincture diluted with water) and sometimes given internally.
- Ear—Hard hearing from Concussion.
- Epistaxis.
- Nosebleed; preceded by tingling; from mechanical causes; whooping cough; typhus.
- Toothache after operation, plugging, etc.
- Putrid smell from mouth.
- Eructation; frequent; empty; bitter.
- Vomiting of dark red coagula, mouth bitter; general soreness. After injuries.
- Foul belching.
- Dyspepsia. Prolapsus ani.
- Offensive flatus; smelling like rotten eggs.
- Stool involuntary during sleep (also urine). Fever. Apoplexy. etc.
- Dysentery with ischuria, or tenesmus of neck of bladder with fruitless urging.
- Most marked indication is long intervals between stools, namely from four to six hours.
- Bladder affections after mechanical injuries.
- Tenesmus from spasms of neck of bladder.
- Constant urging while urine passes involuntarily in drops.
- Frequent attempts to urinate.
- Has to wait a long time for urine to pass.
- Retention of urine from exertion.
- Ischuria with dysentery.
- Involuntary urination at night during sleep. Apoplexy. Typhus, etc.
- Urine brown with lateritous sediment.
- Haematuria from mechanical causes.
- Urine thick, with much pus and some blood globules, but no tubes. Nephritis.
- Urine very acid, with increase of specific gravity.
- Penis and testis swollen purple-red; after injuries.
- Phymosis from friction; parts bruised and much swollen.
- Female—Threatened abortion from falls, shocks, etc.; ner-vous, exited; feel bruised.

- Soreness of parts after labour; prevents haemorrhage.
- Sore nipples.
- Asthma from fatty degeneration of heart.
- Whooping cough; child cries before paroxysm as though in fear of soreness it will cause, cough causes blood-shot eyes, nosebleed, expectoration of foaming blood, or clots of blood.
- Haemorrhage after mechanical injuries; slight spitting of black, thick, viscid blood, or bright red, frothy blood, mixed with mucus and coagula.
- Haemoptysis. (Coughing of blood)
- Pleurisy after mechanical injuries; must continually change position, bed feels so hard.
- Pneumothorax from external injuries.
- "Strain of the heart" from violent running.
- Fatty degeneration of heart.
- Pulse at rest below 60, after moving above 120. Nephritis.
- Articulations and cartilaginous connections of chest feel as if beaten, when moving, breathing, or coughing.
- Hygroma patellae.
- A splinter ran deep into sole a month ago, producing a great deal of proud flesh, came out after inner and outer use.
- Paralytic pains in all joints during motion, as if bruised.
- Complaints from exertion; hoarse, overusing voice; palpitation; fornication, lame; paralysis; bruised feeling; sciatica; weary, faint; retained urine, nosebleed.
- Head feels too hot for him, body feels chilly and cold, between frequent attacks of violent convulsion. After Acon.
- General sinking of strength; he can scarcely move a limb. Typhus.
- While answering, falls into a deep sleep before finishing. Typhus.
- Frequent violent attacks of chill. Nephritis.
- Chilly, with heat and redness of one check.
- Head feels too hot to him, body chilly and cold; < between frequent attacks of convulsion.
- Malaria intermittents.
- Traumatic Fever.
- Typhoid conditions.

- Putrid Fever.
- Heat in oft-repeated short attacks.
- Concussion and contusions.
- Burrowing pus, not painful.
- Prevents suppuration.
- Hypersonic is rather a contra-indication for Arn.
- Septicaemia; tendency to typhoid forms.
- Myalgia; particularly after over-exertion.
- Gout and rheumatism.
- Inflammation of skin and cellular tissue; tender on pressure.
- Everything on which he lies seems too hard.
- Sprain, with much swelling, bluish redness, intense soreness.
- After bruises with blunt instruments. Iritis.
- Concussion; falls; mechanical injuries.
- Contusions with lacerations.
- Stings of bees or wasps; splinters.
- Compound Fracture, and their profuse suppuration.
- Pressure; aching in epigastrium < ; liver sensitive, spleen sore; stitches in chest >.
- Mechanical injuries; concussion of brain while there are unconsciousness, parole or drowsiness; weak intermitting pulse; cold surface and other indications or depressed vitality from shock; threatened abortion; ovarian troubles; orchitis; mastitis, etc.
- Many small toils painful, one after another; extremely sore.

  Acon.,

  Ipec.,

  Verat.-after Apis. in Hydrocephalus.
- Complementary to Acon.

ARSENICUM ALBUM

I. Introduction (Cow-92)

Synonym: Arsenious Acid.
Preparation: Trituration, Hahnemann's provings but not published in MMP. He included in 1816 in IInd volume, since people cried him out as a poison doctor (Hering in Pierce-279).

II. General Analysis (Cow.)

Ars. is an irritant poison and has specific action almost upon every organ tissue and secretion of the body. It acts directly upon blood composition, upon the tissue and upon nervous system. The condition produced is one of asthenia (weakness), leading to exhaustion of vital power. The leading characteristics of Ars. (Pierce-Plain Talks) are— Periodicity, Irritability, Anguish, Prostation and Restlessness, Thirst, Burning pains, Relief from heat, fear of incurability. Neuralgic headache < night.

III. Suited to (Allen-49)

Great prostration with rapid sinking of the vital forces, fainting. Mentally restless, but physically too weak to move, can't rest in any place. Burning pains, as if hot coals applied to parts (Anthrac.), > heat, hot drinks or hot applications.

IV. Clinical (Clarke-I-177)

Abscess, Acne rosacea, Alcoholism, Amenorrhoea, Anaemia, Aphthae, Asthma, Atrophy, Bronchitis, Brow ague, Caecum-affections of, Cancer, Cancrum oris, Carbuncles, Cholera Asistica, Cholera, Colds, Coldness, Commissures-soreness of, Cough, Coxalgia, Croup, Dandruff, Delirium tremens, Depression of spirits, Diarrhoea, Diphtheria,

Dropsy, Duodenum, Dyspepsia, Ears-affections of, Eczema, Endometritis, Enteric fever, Epithelioma, Erysipelas, Eye affections, Face-eruption on, Fainting, Fever, Gangrene, Gastric ulcer, Gastritis, Gastrodynia, Glandular swellings, Gout, Hay-asthma, Headache, Heart affections, Hectic, Herpes zoster, Hodgkin's disease, Hydrothorax, Hypochondriasis, Ichthyosis, Indigestion, Intermittent fever, Irritation, Jaundice, Kidney-diseases of, Leucorrhoea, Lichen, Lips-eruption round; Lips-epithelioma of, Locomotor ataxy, Lung affections, Lupus, Malignant pustule, Measles, Melancholia, Menstruation disordered, Miliary eruption, Morphoea, Myelitis, Nails diseased, Nettlerash, Neuralgia, Neuritis, Noma pudendi, Numbness, Peritonitis, Perityphlitis, Pityriasis, Plethora, Pleurisy, Pleurodynia, Pneumonia, Psoriasis, Purpura, Pyaemia, Pyelitis, Remittent fever, Rheumatic gout, Rheumatism, Rickets, Ringworm, Scald-head, Scarlatina, Sciatica, Scrofulous affections, Sea-bathing-effects of, Sea-sickness, Shivering, Stomach-affections of, Strains, Suppuration, Thirst, Throat sore, Tobacco-habit, Tongue-affections of, Trachea-affections of, Traumatic fever, Typhus, Ulcer, Vomiting, Whooping-cough, Worms, Wounds, Yellow fever.

V. **Symptoms-General** (Nash-87)

1. Great anguish and restlessness, driving from place to place.
2. Great sudden prostration, sinking of vital force.
3. Intense burning pains.
4. Intense thirst, drinks often but little, as cold water disagrees.
5. Dyspnoea < on motion, esp. ascending.
6. Vomiting and stool simultaneous, < after eating or drinking.
7. Modalities: < in cold air from cold things, cold applications, and 1-3 AM Movement. > by warm air or room, hot application, by sweat.

VI. **Symptoms-Particular** (Nash-87-94)

1. Alimentary canal, most profoundly affected.

(a) Mouth-lips dry cracked, throat / tongue dry, Mouth-dry ulcerated

(b) Thirst-intense, can take only a little water at a time, but frequently.

Ars.,

Bry.-intense-large quantity of water at long interval

Puls.-No thirst, dry mouth

(c) Stomach pains-cold food/drink disagrees. Covers all problems and affections ranging along whole length of the canal, with Ars. symptoms.

2. Respiratory organs

(a) Nasal coryza-acute (All. c., Merc. c.) more burning.

(b) Respiration (affections of the lung) that leads to fluent discharge corrodes nose and lips, wheezing, cough with frothy expectoration. Can't lie down- Ars.,

Carb. v.-must sit up to breathe.

3. Great Prostation

Ars.-Out of proportion, Another characteristic besides prostration,

General weakness, yet he wants to move for relief constantly.

Mur. ac.
Carb. v. } utter absence of such show of life.

Ars.—weakness is general, not local or as shown below:

Particular weakness:

Phos. ac.
Stan.
Sul. } In chest

Phos.-in abdomen

Ign.
Hydras.
Sep. } In the stomach

4. Skin dry, scaly and always burning. Suppressed skin eruption. Suppressed eczema. One of the best remedies for retrocadent (suppressed) exanthemeta and eczema etc.

5. Restlessness. Tosses about, driving from place to place for relief, which he does not get. Later stages of illness, when he becomes weak. Mental restlessness-has attack of anxiety, even when there is no pain, he changes places. He has fear of death, but not like Acon. Fear, but of anxiety that it is useless to take medicine.
   Acon., Arn., Rhus t.
6. Burner-anywhere, everywhere.
   Ars.-> heat, warm room, warm application on the affected part. < midnight
   Sul.-alone out ranks it as burner.
   Sec.-burning but part / body cold (objective), heat intolerable.
7. Fluent Coryza
   Ars.-excoriating nasal discharge>hot application.
   All. c.-Excoriating tears, bland nasal discharge.
   Merc. c.
8. Periodicity
   Ars.-1-2 AM / PM
   Lyc.-4-8 PM.
   Nux. v.-3-4 AM.
   Nat. m.-11 AM.
   Sul.-5 AM. 11 AM.
   Cedr.-Same time every day.
9. Typhoid Fever
   Ars., (intermittent fever abo)
   Mur. ac.,
   Carb. v..

VII. Black Letter Symptoms
(Tyler 98-100)

- Very violent delirium, especially at night, with great restlessness.
- Her desire exceeds her need (eats and drinks more than is good for her; walks, further than she needs to do).
- Despairs and weeps; imagines no one can help him, that he must die; is cold and chilly, and afterwards generally weak.

- Anguish, Excessive anguish.
- Anguish and despair—driving from one place to another, for relief.
- With great anguish he turns and tosses to and fro in his bed.
- Restlessness and anxiety. Throwing himself from side to side.
- Anxiety at 3 O' clock after midnight.
- Violent anxiety at 3 O' clock in the night; he felt hot as if he would vomit.
- Dread of death coming on suddenly when alone.
- The greatest fear and anguish (sees ghosts day and night).
- (Great heaviness in the head; it goes off in the open air; but returns as soon as he enters the room).
- Burning in eyes.
- Eyelids oedematous, often completely closing the eyes.
- Corrosive tears, making cheeks and eyelids sore.
- Excoriating discharge from nostrils.
- Watery discharge from nose, went off in the open air; watery nasal discharge causes smarting and burning, as if nostrils were made sore by it.
- Face expressive of genuine mental agony.
- Deathly colour of face. Pale, yellow cachectic look.
- Swelling of face, or sunken face.
- (Tongue furred, with a red streak down middle) and redness of tip.
- Dryness of tongue.
- Dry and brown coated tongue.
- Feeling of great dryness in mouth with violent thirst; drinks little at a time.
- Burning in mouth along the pharynx and in the pit of the stomach.
- Loathing of food.
- Excessive thirst: drinking did not refresh him.
- Excessive thirst; he drinks much, but little at a time.
- Long-lasting hiccough at the hour when the fever ought to come.
- Nausea.

- Vomiting violent and incessant and exited by any substance taken into the stomach.
- Even water is immediately thrown off the stomach.
- Vomiting every time after drinking.
- The vomiting brings no relief.
- Frequent vomiting with apprehensions of death.
- Anxiety in the pit of the stomach.
- Burning in the stomach.
- Violent burning pains in the stomach.
- In the stomach fearful burning pains.
- Swollen abdomen.
- Distension and pain in abdomen.
- Pains in abdomen with unbearable anxiety: with intolerable anguish.
- Burning pains in abdomen.
- The evacuations excoriated the skin about anus.
- Burning like fire at anus.
- Purging and extreme coldness of extremities. Constipation.
- Burning in urethra during micturation.
- Scanty emission and burning during micturation.
- Involuntary micturation.
- Frequent oppressive shortness of breath in every position of the body, causing anxiety. (Chest).
- Oppression-want of breath-a nocturnal asthma makes him spring up at midnight.
- Difficult breathing, with great anguish.
- Oppression or breath when walking fast.
- The heart beats are irritable.
- Palpitation. Irregular palpitation of the heart, but so violent at night that he imagines he hears it.
- Palpitation of heart and tremulous weakness after stool: he has to lie down.
- Quick, weak, and irregular pulse.
- Loss of strength in the small of the back.
- Excessive weakness and exhaustion of the limbs, obliging him to lie down.
- Uneasiness in lower limbs, he cannot lie still at night, and had to change the position of his feet all the time or to walk about, to get relief.

- Very great restlessness, so that she could not lie quite a minute, restlessness and anxiety. Throwing himself from side to side.
- The slightest paroxysm of pain is accompanied with an excessive sinking of strength, obliging him to lie down.
- He is so weak that he is scarcely able to walk: feels he will fall over; scarcely able to walk across the room without sinking down.
- Continued weakness and prostration.
- Great weariness after a meal.
- Faintness and insensibility.
- Faint, anxious, weak, early in the morning.
- Burning pains, especially in the inner organs, skin and ulcers.
- Eruption round mouth, burning and painful.
- Itch, increased by scratching.
- Burning pain in the ulcers-as from glowing coals.
- Burning like fire around the ulcer.
- Burning itching of body.
- Startings when falling asleep in the evening.
- After midnight (from 3 O'clock) she tosses about and sleeps only at times.
- Shuddering when walking in the open air.
- Shuddering without thirst.
- Fever at 2 O'clock in the night.
- Typhus-like fever with extreme restlessness.
- Burning heat internally.
- Feels as if burning up internally.
- Feeling of heat with anxiety, after midnight.
- Cold, clammy sweat.

ARUM TRIPHYLLUM

I. Introduction (Clarke-I-200)

Common Name: Indian Turnip.
Natural Order: Araceae
Preperation: Tincture of fresh tuber or corm.

II. Suited to (Allen-51)

Persons who pick and bore into raw bleeding surfaces though very painful; scream with pain but keep up the boring (in Diphtheria, Typhoid). Children refuse food and drink on account of soreness of throat and mouth (Merc. c.), are sleepless.

III. Clinical (Clarke-I-200)

Brain-inflammation of, Clergyman's sore throat, Delirium, Diphtheria, Glandular swellings, Headache, Jaw-joint painful, Mouth sore, Scarlatina, Tongue cracked, Typhoid fever, Voice hoarse.

IV. Symptoms-General (Nash-385)

1. Raw, red, bloody surface of lips, nose, buccal cavity; patients pick and bore into them incessantly, through they are so sore and painful.
2. Hoarseness, with changing voice when exciting it; from high to low and vice versa.
3. Discharges generally very acrid or corrosive; exceptionally bland.

V. Symptoms-Particular (Nash-385)

1. Raw, red bloody surface of lips, mouth and nose. Whenever in any disease this red, raw condition of mouth, nose, lips, at which the patient bores and picks, Arum. t. is the medicine.
2. Hoarseness, with changing voice-high to low and vice versa. (Larynx and Bronchia) the voice breaks, sore throat of clergymen and opera singers.

   Arg. n.,
   Arn.,
   Caust.,
   Sel.,
   Phos.

ASAFOETIDA

I. Introduction (Clarke-I-203)

Common Name: Italian Grass
Natural Order.: Gramineae.
Preperation: Tincture of root sprouts.

II. Clinical (Clark-I-203)

Asthma, Bone disease, Chorea, Diarrhoea, Dyspepsia, Flatulence, Headache, Heart affections, Hypersensitiveness, Hysteria, Iritis, Lactation disordered, Mercury-effects of, Neuralgia, Obesity, Orbita neuralgia, Ozaena, Syphilis, Tympanites, Ulcer, Whitlow.

III. Black Letter Symptoms (Tyler-102)

- Pressive pain in forehead, from within outwards.
- Nervous headache of hysterical or scrofulous people.
- Nocturnal throbbing pain in and around eye and HEAD.
- Extensive superficial ulceration of cornea, with burning, sticking or pressing, from within out. Better rest, pressure, open air. Numbness round EYE.
- Discharge of very offensive matter from NOSE; with Caries of the bones.
- Swelling of lower lip.
- Sensation of a ball rising in throat from STOMACH to oesophagus.
- Flatus passing upwards; none down.
- Heat in spleen and ABDOMEN.
- Watery liquid STOOLS of the most disgusting smell.
- Pains in abdomen and discharge of foetid flatus.
- Watery stools of disgusting odour, profuse and greenish.

- URINE warm and of a pungent, ammoniacal smell.
- Spasmodic tightness of CHEST, as if lungs could not fully expand. Asthmatic feeling in trachea, dry cough; spasmodic dyspnoea as if lungs could not be fully expanded.
- Pain and tenderness TIBIA, almost unbearable at night.
- Nervous PALPITATION with small pulse, from over-exertion or suppression of discharges.
- Hysteria, with much trouble about throat or oesophagus; well marked globus; spasm of lungs, etc.
- Nervous affections after suppressed discharges.
- Nervous people.

AURUM METALLICUM

I. Introduction (Cow-116)

Synonym: Aurum Metallicum.
Common Name: Metallic Gold.
Preparation: Trituration of precipitated metal.

As a medicine, at least in Europe, Hahnemann proved Gold in 1818, and declared its mighty curative powers. Reason given in MMP-I for not treating gold as medicine was that even most intense heat could not alter it, then how could mild heat of stomach (Pierce-pg. 296).

II. General Analysis (Cow.)

It affects osseous (semi circular canals-ear) and glandular systems prominently, nasal and palatine (to palate) bones. Besides its local action the peculiar features are—Despondent melancholy with suicidal tendency.

III. Suited to (Allen-55)

Sanguine, ruddy people, with black hair and eye, lively, restless, anxious about future. Old people, weak vision, tired of life. For constitutions broken down by bad effects of mercury and syphilis. Pining boys: low spirited, lifeless, weak memories, testes undeveloped, lacking in 'boyish go'. Constantly dwelling on suicide (Naja); but afraid to die (Nux. v.).

IV. Clinical (Clarke-I-224)

Alcohol-effects of, Amenorrhoea, Angina pectoris, Asthma, Bone affections, Breath offensive, Corpulency, Depression, Ears-affections of, Erethism, Erysipelas, Eye affections, Fever, Gonorrhoea, Haemorrhage, Haemorrhoids, Hemiopia, Hydrocele, Jaundice, Leucorrhoea, Locomotor ataxy, Melancholy, Melanosis, Mercurial poisoning, Naso-pharyngeal catarrh, Night-terrors, Ozaena, Paralysis, Phthisis, Pining boys, Scrofula, Smell disordered, Syphilis, Testicles-affections of; undeveloped, Tongue-nodules on, Tumours, Uterus-induration of, Vertigo, Vision disordered.

V. **Symptoms-General** (Nash-291)

1. Wants to commit suicide; thinks he is no good in the world.
2. Nodes and bone pains, Caries and Necrosis with great depression of mind.
3. Abuse of Mercury, in Syphilis, in massive doses.

VI. **Symptoms-Particular** (Nash-291)

1. Deepest gloom and tendency to commit suicide
   Aur m., Naja., Nux. v.
2. Carries of long bones (Syphilitic mercurial affections)
   Aur. m.,
   Fluor. ac.,
   Angust., (In nasal catarrh and ulcer-before the actual carries)
3. Hemiopia (Half sight)
   Aur. m.-sees only lower.
   Lyc.,
   Lithic. a } sees only left half of objects.
4. Bone pains (Periosteal affection) (One of the best remedies)
   Aur. m.,
   Kali i.,
   Asa.,
   Merc. c.
5. In women-womb trouble, prolapsus from the very weight of the organs.
6. In men-liver troubles.
7. Nasal troubles-of great use in Catarrh or Ozena, also of the Mastoid process.

VII. Black Letter Symptoms
(Tyler-109-110)

- Disgust of life, suicidal tendency.
- Despondent melancholy. Hopelessness.
- Great anguish increasing into self-destruction.
- Anxious palpitation and desire to commit suicide.
- Peevish and vehement: least contradiction excites wrath.
- Moroseness; indisposed to talk.
- All daylong good humour; talkative and contented with himself (alternating action).
- Heat and anger, quite forgets himself with quarrelling.
- Rush of blood to HEAD.
- Tearing pressures-left forehead, left crown, right side of crown.
- Pressure from within outwards in EYES: worse when touched.
- Tension in eyes interferes with vision.
- Can distinguish nothing distinctly, because he sees everything double and one object seems to run into another: tensive pain worse when he fixed his eyes on something, less severe when he closes them.
- Half-sight-as if the upper half of vision were covered with a dark body- upper objects remain invisible.
- He cannot get air through the NOSE, for ulcerated, agglutinated, painful nostrils, Soreness both nostrils.
- Right nasal bone and adjoining part of upper jaw painful to touch.
- Tickling internally in alae nasi.
- Syphilitic ulcers-Palate and Throat.
- Tensive pain in hypogastrium just below navel and on both sides lumbar regions, with feeling of fullness, and with call to stool.
- Pinching pain in hypogastrium, now here, now there.
- Grumbling and rumbling in ABDOMEN.
- Discharge of much foetid flatus.
- Discomfort in hypogastrium, as if wanted to go to stool, esp. after a meal.

- Affections of genitalia: Uterus prolapsed and indurated.
- Extreme tightness (CHEST): difficulty of breathing at night.
- Tightness of chest, also when sitting and not moving: always takes a deep breath and cannot get enough air.
- Great weight on Chest: esp. heavy weight on sternum.
- Violent beating of the heart.
- Awakened by BONE pains-suffering so great he despairs-does not want to live.
- Pain in knees as if they were tightly bound.
- Remarkable ebullition in the BLOOD (as if it boiled in the blood vessels).
- Sulky.
- Frightful dreams at night.

BAPTISIA TINCTORIA

I. Introduction (Cow-122)

Synonym: Baptisia Tinctoria.
Natural Order: Leguminosæ.
Common Name: Wild Indigo.
Habitat: A perennial herb growing in dry poor soil throughout USA
Preparation: Tincture from fresh roots.
It was proved in 1857 by Dr. Thomson (Pierce-299).

II. General Analysis (Cow.)

Acts esp. upon blood having a disorganising and decomposing influence. Affects mucous membranes of esp. mouth, throat, and intestines; also motor and sensory nerves, giving rise to both prostration and paralysis of motion and sensation. Its chief indications are—bruised and weary feeling; Brain-fag in low fever; lassitude; delusions of dismemberment.

III. Suited to (Allen-57)

Lymphatic temperament. Aversion to mental exertion. Stupor, falls asleep while answering or being spoken to. Great prostration-feels body scattered about the bed, aversion to mental exertion, painless sore throat, can swallow liquid only (Baryt. c.). Part rested upon feels sore and bruised. (Pyr., Arn.)

IV. Clinical (Clarke-I-243)

Abortion threatened, Apoplexy, Appendicitis, Biliousness, Brain softening, Cancer, Consumption, Diphtheria, Dysentery, Enteric fever, Eye affections, Gall-Bladder affections, Gastric fever, Headache-bilious, Hectic fever,

Hysteria, Influenza, Mumps, Oesophagus-constriction of, Plague, Relapsing fever, Sewer-gas poisoning, Shivering, Stomatitis, Tabes mesenterica, Tinea capitis, Tongue ulcerated, Typhus, Variola, Worms.

V. **Symptoms-General** (Nash-257)

1. Mind confused; as if drunk; cannot collect himself; feels scattered about, cannot get pieces together.
2. Face dark dusky; eyes bleared, besotted expression.
3. Mouth ulcerated, with foul smell; or dry, tongue dry in a streak down the centre.
4. Abdomen sensitive in right iliac region, with rumbling. Stool loose, and urine with all other discharges; very offensive.
5. Awakes with oppressed feeling, must have more air.
6. Great prostration with aching and soreness all over. Great typhoid remedy.
7. Can swallow liquids only; least solid food gags.
8. In whatever position the patient lies, the part rested upon feels sore and bruised. (Lach., Pyr.).

VI. **Symptoms-Particular** (Nash-258)

1. Typhoid. A Typhoid remedy, comes after Gels stage. Indicators are-great nervousness, chilliness, aching pains all over, drowsy, face and eyes give besotted appearance. Grows week. Feels scattered around the bed. Tongue streaked down the middle, at first white than brown.
2. Bowels-rumbling, offensive discharges, ilio-coecal region sensitive to touch, all discharges very offensive.

VII. **Black Letter Symptoms** (Tyler-115)

- Stupor; falls asleep while being spoken to, or answering; heavy sleep until roused; wakes only to fall asleep again in the midst of his answer, which he vainly endeavours to finish.
- Confusion of ideas. Confusion as if drunk.
- She cannot go to sleep, because cannot get herself together.

- Feels scattered about, and tosses about to get the pieces together. Aversion to mental exertion. Indisposed to think; mind seems weak.
- Dull bruised feeling in occiput.
- Face sallow: dark-red; with a besotted expression; flushed; dusky.
- Sordes on teeth and lips: tongue ulcerated.
- Foetid odour of mouth (Merc. c.)
- Fauces dark-red: dark, putrid ulcers-unusual absence of pain.
- Tonsils and soft palate swollen; not accompanied by pain.
- Can swallow liquids only. The least food gags.
- Oesophagus feels constricted from above down to stomach.
- Paralysis of organs of deglutition (Gels.)
- Right iliac region sensitive.
- Abdominal muscles sore on pressure, with acute intermitting pain.
- Foetid, exhausting diarrhoea, causing excoriation.
- Drowsy; stupid; delirious stupor.
- Cerebral forms of fever.
- Typhoid and cerebral forms of fever, with delirium, drowsiness.
- Feeling head or limbs, scattered, etc. Involuntary scanty stool, difficult breathing.
- Prostration with disposition of fluids to decompose.
- Discharge and exhalations foetid; breath stools, urine, sweat, ulcers.
- Ulceration, especially of mouth; also with tendency to putrescence.

BARYTA CARBONICA

I. Introduction (Cow-125)

Synonym: Carbon of Barium
Preparation: Trituration.

II. General Analysis (Cow.)

Its most characteristic effect is upon glandular system esp. glands of the throat and neck. It is a remedy adapted to extremes of life; for infancy with too low and imperfect development; for old age with too rapid deterioration and too early. Not as old as he looks. Baryt. c. was proved by Hahnemann with 290 symptoms (Chronic Diseases-I).

III. Suited to (Allen-58)

Complaints of first and second childhood, psoric or tubercular. Memory deficient-Scrofulous, dwarfish children who do not grow (grow too rapidly-Calc. c.); Cornea opaque. Child physically, mentally weak.

IV. Clinical (Clarke-I-248)

Aneurism, Apoplexy, Atrophy, Baldness, Brain-affection of, Cysts, Foot-sweat, Glandular swellings, Haemorrhoids, Heart affections, Memory defective, Oesophagus-spasm of, Panaris, Paralysis, Parotitis, Prostate enlarged, Quinsy, Throat sore, Tonsil enlarged, Tumours, Warts, Wens.

V. Symptoms-General (Nash-352)

1. Mental and physical weakness; both ends of life; don't grow. Almost imbecile (children) feeble and tottering; childish and thoughtless (old age); loss of memory.

2. Tonsils inflame, swell and suppurate repeatedly, on every cold exposure; chronic hypertrophy afterwards. Glands swell, infiltrate, hypertrophy; neck, parotids, sub-maxillary, groin, lymphatics, in the abdomen; hypertrophy, sometimes suppuration.
3. Offensive foot sweats; toes and soles get sore; throat affection after checked foot-sweat.
4. Great sensitiveness to cold.

VI. **Symptoms-Particular** (Nash-352)

1. Anti scrofulous, Quinsy (Tonsil), Mental, Physical weakness.
2. Like Calc. c., a constitutional medicine. Complaints of dwarfish children, mind and body weak, docile (infantile and senile), grow inclined to glandular swellings. Defective growth is physical and mental both.

Sil.-Profuse sweat on head. Baryt. c.-No sweat on head. Sil.-Strong will power. Bry.-Weak will power. Abrot., Nat. m.	Emaciation of the rest of the body while abdomen is greatly enlarged. Voracious appetite yet poor growth. Sil. and Baryt. c. (resemblance), offensive sweat on feet; head disproportionately large than body; < damp change in weather and sensitive to cold about head.

3. Affinity for Throat (esp. Tonsils) worse least exposure to cold,

Baryt. c.-tonsils greatly inflamed, swollen, and suppurate, on least exposure to cold.

Psor.-(In Quinsy after Baryt. c.)

Lach.,

Lyc.,

Phyt.

BELLADONNA

I. Introduction (Cow-129)

Synonym: Atropa Belladonna.
Natural Order: Solanaceae.
Common Name: Deadly Nightshade.
Habitat: Herbaceous perennial plant, native of Europe.
Preparation: Tincture from entire fresh plant.

It was proved by Hahnemann who recorded 1440 symptoms (MMP).

II. General Analysis (Cow.)

Its centre of action is the cerebrum from where it affects the entire organism. Sensorium is prominently affected causing delirium, illusion, hallucinations, stupor and insomnia. It acts as a powerful irritant to the entire nervous system, producing congestion and in consequence general hyperaesthesia of both sensory and motor nerves. Senses become acute. Spasm, or convulsion in voluntary muscle system. Skin hot shining red. Mucous membranes, especially are of eyes, mouth, throat and genito-urinary organs. Most characteristic expressions are—flushed face hard and bounding pulse, suddenness, local inflammations and wild delirium.

III. Suited to (Allen-59)

Bilious, plethoric constitutions-well and lively, when ill violent. Women and children with light hair, blue eyes, fair complexion, sensitive, nervous. Great debility to take cold, uncovering head, from hair cut, tonsils inflamed from cold air (Acon., Hep. s., Rhus t.), takes cold from exposure to feet (Con., Cupr., Sil.). Convulsion-during teething with fever (without fever Mag. phos.), Rush of blood to head and face (Amyl nit., Glon., Meli.), Vertigo when stooping or rising after stooping (Bry.), Headache with red face, throbbing with carotids (Meli.).

IV. Clinical (Clarke-I-256)

Abscess, Acne, Amaurosis, Apoplexy, Bladder weakness, Boils, Brain-affections of, Bronchial glands-disease of, Carbuncles, Colic, Constipation, Convulsions, Cough, Croup, Delirium tremens, Depression, Diarrhoea, Dysentery, Ear affections , Enteric fever, Epilepsy, Erysipelas, Erythema, Excitement, Eye affections, Fear-effects of, Glandular swellings, Goitre, Gout, Haemorrhoids, Headache, Heart affections, Hydrocephalus, Hydrophobia, Hyperoemia, Influenza, Kidney-affections of, Lung affections, Malignant pustule, Mania, Measles, Meningitis, Menstruation, Mouth affections, Mumps, Neuralgia, Nose affections, Nyctalopia, Nymphomania, Paralysis, Parametritis, Perichondritis, Perimetritis, Peritonitis, Phlegmasia alba dolens, Pleurisy, Pneumogastric paralysis, Pneumonia, Pregnancy-affections of, Puerperal mania, Rheumatism, Roseola, Scarlatina, Sensitiveness, Sleep disordered, Smell disordered, Strangury, Taste disordered, Tenesmus, Testicles-affections of, Thirst, Throat sore, Tongue-affections of, Tuberculosis, Ulcer, Uterine affections, Vaccinia, Vertigo, Whooping-cough, Worm fever.

V. Symptoms-General (Nash-99)

1. All acute inflammatory diseases present prominent head symptoms, pain, red puffed face, throbbing carotids and delirium, and spasms, or jerks and twitching.
2. Eyes staring, red, blood-shot: pupils first contracted, then greatly dilated.
3. Mouth and throat very dry, red sometimes greatly swollen; all mucous surfaces correspondingly dry and hot.
4. Pains appear suddenly-after a while disappear as suddenly as they came.
5. Skin very red and hot, fairly radiates heat; burns the hand touching it, but sweats on covered parts.
6. Several inflammations which streak out in radii from a centre.
7. Modalities: < after 3 PM or after midnight from

uncovering, or draft of air, and lying down; > from covering and head high.

8. Great liability to take cold; sensitive to draft of air, especially when uncovering the head; From having the hair cut (Hep. s.), Tonsils swell after riding in a cold wind (Acon.)
9. Imagines he sees ghosts, hideous faces, and various insects (Stram.); black animals, dogs and wolves.
10. Abdomen tender, distended < least jar, even the bed; obliged to walk with great care for fear of a jar.
11. Pain in right ilio-caecal region, < by slightest touch, even the bed covers.
12. Pressing downwards, as if the contents of abdomen would issue from the vulva; < standing and sitting erect; worse mornings (compare Lil. t., Mur. p., Sep.).
13. Tongue: Red and dry, with red edges and white coating in the middle; papillae bright and prominent, like Scarletina (Acon., Ant. tar.), offensive putrid taste in throat when eating or drinking, although food tastes natural.

VI. Symptoms-Particular (Nash-100-105)

1. *Delirium Trio*

   Bell., Hyo., Stram.
2. *A head remedy-Bell.-Blood seems rushing to head* (Amyl nit.,Glon., Meli.) Head hot while extremities are cold, Eyes blood red, Face-purple red.
3. Ist stage inflammations (Local) Anywhere if it comes—
   a. Suddenly and rapid course
   b. Red and painful part
   c. Throbbing

   Merc. c., Hep. s., Tarent. cub. and Bell. for local inflammations.
4. *Diseases of children*—child well one minute and sick the next, child very hot, next with red face and semi-stupor, jumps in sleep, as if it might go into spasms.

   Cham.-Bell. vies with.

   Cina.-sudden and intense onset of fever as in Bell.
5. PAINS in {
   Bell.-appear suddenly, disappear suddenly.
   Stan.-appear gradually, disappear gradually
   Sul.a-appear slowly, disappear suddenly.

6. *Headache*

Throbbing-due to congestion of blood in the head.

< stooping forward
< bending downward } general characteristic of Bell. pains.
< lying down

7. *Throat.* Bell. has great affinity for the throat.

Bell. —red, inflamed, sense of constriction, burning dryness.

Saba. —burning dryness.

Lyss. —sense of constriction, constant desire to swallow to remove it.

8. *Abdomen.*

(a) Tender, < least jar in walking, stepping, even in bed or chair, upon or sits lies.

(b) Pressure downwards as if contents of abdomen would go through vulva. < mornings. (Lil. t., Sep.). In Bell., with this pressure as if the back would break.

9. Sleepy but can't, moans during sleep.
10. *Cold in head when uncovering, cutting hair* (Sil.)

Ant. c.-after river bath.

Glon.-can't bear hat.

11. Skin uniform, smooth, shining, scarlet, redness, redness of skin-so hot that it imparts a burning sensation to one who touches for some time.
12. Convulsion with other Bell. symptoms are very frequently found.

VII. Black Letter Symptoms (Tyler-120-123)

- Inclination to bite those around them.
- She attempted to bite and strike her attendants, broke into fits of laughter, gnashed her teeth. The head was hot, the face red, the look wild and fierce.
- Inclination to bite those around him and to tear everything about him to pieces.
- Raging, violent fury. Furious delirium. She pulled at the hair of the bystanders.

- Such fury (with burning heat of the body, and open, staring, immovable eyes) that she had to be held constantly, lest she would attack someone; and when thus held, so that she could not move, she spat continually at those about her.
- The face was red, the head hot, the look wild and staring: pupils dilated: the arteries of the neck and head visibly pulsating.
- In the evening he was seized with such violent delirium that it required three men to confine him. His face was livid, his eyes injected and protruding; the pupils strongly dilated; the carotid arteries pulsating most violently; a full hard frequent pulse, with loss of power to swallow.
- Great intolerance of light and noise.
- He sought continually to spring out of bed. When put to bed he sprang out again in delirium, talked constantly, laughed out, and exhibited complete loss of consciousness, did not know his own parents.
- Rush of blood to the head: pulsation of cerebral arteries, and a throbbing in the interior of the head. Very intense headache.
- The pains in the head are aggravated by noise, motion, when moving the eyes, by contact.
- Afraid to cough on account of the increase of pain it causes.
- Pressive headache, especially in forehead.
- Painful pressure in head, especially lower part of forehead directly above the nose, intolerable on stepping or treading.
- Three violent stabs, forehead to occiput, whereupon all previous headache suddenly disappears.
- Violent throbbing in brain from behind forwards and towards both sides; throbbing ends on the surface in painful shootings.
- Jerking headache, violent on walking quickly or going rapidly upstairs. At every step it seemed as if the brain rose and fell in the forehead; the pain ameliorated by pressing strongly on the forehead. (The only "better for pressure" of Belladona ?).

- Stabbing as if with a knife from temple to temple.
- The head is so sensitive that the least contact gives her pain.
- Eyes projecting and sparking: pupils dilated.
- A startling look. Distorted, with redness and swelling of face.
- Eyes dry; motion attended with sense of dryness and stiffness.
- Burning heat in eyes.
- Dilated pupils: dilated and immovable.
- Everything he sees looks red.
- Great sensitiveness of smell.
- Great redness of the face: glowing red face, with inexpressible pains in the head. Face, neck and chest much swollen.
- Tumefaction and redness of face and lips.
- Spasmodic action of the muscles of the face.
- Convulsive movements of face, with distortion of mouth.
- The tongue and palate dark red. Dryness of throat and difficult swallowing.
- Dryness of tongue and throat, so great as to interfere with speech, Dryness of fauces most distressing.
- During deglutition, feeling in throat as if it were too narrow, as if nothing would pass properly.
- Scrapping raw sensation of epiglottis: raw and sore.
- Nausea.
- Long-lasting painfulness of the whole abdomen, as if it were all raw and sore.
- Excessive tenderness of abdomen, which cannot bear the slightest touch.
- Violent cutting pressure in hypogastrium, now here, now there.
- Retention of urine, which only passes drop by drop.
- Badly smelling haemorrhage from the uterus.
- Violent pressing and urging towards the sexual organs as if everything would fall out there.
- Menses too soon and very profuse, of thick, decomposed, dark-red blood.
- Catarrh or cough with coryza.

- Painful dryness in larynx.
- Larynx as if inflamed and swollen.
- Hoarseness.
- Hollow, hoarse cough.
- Pulse full and quick.
- Various symptoms of extremities.
- Thighs and legs, as if bruised all over, as if rotten.
- Shooting and gnawing along the shafts of bones-tearing in joints
- Epileptic Convulsion.
- Every moment wished to get out of bed.
- The boy wished to escape.
- Great irritability and impressiveness of the senses.
- Tastes and smells everything more acutely.
- Taste, sight and hearing keener; mind more easily moved and thoughts more active.
- Excessive nervous excitability with exalted sensibility of all the organs. The least noise, light-annoying.
- Redness of the whole body with quick pulse.
- Redness like Scarlatina of the entire surface of the body.
- Pustules break out on cheeks and nose.
- He starts as if in fright and awakes, when just falling asleep.
- Starts as if in a fright, feeling as if she were falling down deep (Thuj.), which caused her to shudder violently.
- Very restless sleep.
- At night the boy becomes restless, speaks irrationally, and can with difficulty be kept in bed.
- The child tosses about, kicks and quarrels in its sleep.
- Temperature of the head very much increased.
- The skin hot, dry, scarlet, especially intense on face and ears.
- Burning heat within and without.
- Whatever the ailment-headache, fever, inflammation-where there is burning heat, redness, pain that will not bear pressure, jar or motion, think of Belladonna.

BENZOIC ACID

I. Introduction (Cow-140)

Synonym: Benzoic Acidum
Preparation: Pure crystals are dissolved in alcohol.

II. General Analysis (Cow.)

Acts upon urinary organs giving rise to a Uric acid diathesis, affecting joints, tendons. Main characteristic is deep Red colour urine with strong urinous odour.

III. Suited to (Allen-62)

Persons with rheumatic diathesis engrafted on a syphilitic or gonorrhoeal patient. Urine dark brown and odor highly intensified.

IV. Clinical (Clarke)

Asthma, Bladder affections, Bunions, Cracks, Diarrhoea, Enuresis, Eye-tumours of, Ganglion, Gonorrhoea, Gout, Joint affections, Knee-pain in, Rheumatism, Sycosis, Throat sore, Tongue sore, Tonsil enlarged, Ulcer, Urine-disorders of, Wens.

V. Symptoms-Particular (Nash-314)

1. Urine dark brown colour-urinous odour highly intensified.

   Nit. ac.-like horse urine.
   Berb. v.-Turbid deposits.
   Benz. ac.-smells horrible, but no deposits at all.
   Calc. c.-white deposit with offensive smell.
2. Dribbling of urine in old men with enlarged prostate.
3. Rheumatism, quinsy, dropsy, diarrhoea, headache etc. with systems call for it.

4. Arthritis
   Lyc.,
   Lith. c,
   Benz. ac.,
   Berb. v.

BERBERIS VULGARIS

I. Introduction (Cow-141)

Synonym: Berberis Vulgaris.
Natural Order: Berberidaceae.
Common Name: Barberry.
Habitat: Indigenous European plant.
Preparation: Tincture from the bark of fresh root.

It is an old medicine but it was first proved in 1834 by Dr. Hesse of Germany (Pierce-312).

II. General Analysis (Cow.)

Special action upon kidneys and bladder—where it causes shooting pains; upon liver-where it promotes flow of bile, Main Sympton is Pam in the region of kidneys and upon mucous membranes and muscular system.

III. Suited to (Allen-62)

Renal, vesicle symptoms—Pain in the small of the back very sensitive ιo touch in renal region-Pale, earthy complexion, with sunken check, and hollow blue circled eyes. Colic from Gall stones.

IV. Clinical (Clarke-I-280)

Biliary colic, Bilious attack, Bladder affections, Calculi, Duodenum-catarrh of, Dysmenorrhoea, Fever, Fistula, Gall-stones, Gravel, Herpes, Irritation, Jaundice, Joint affections, Knee-pain in, Leucorrhoea, Liver disorder, Lumbago, Ophthalmia, Oxaluria, Polypi, Renal colic, Rheumatism, Sacrum-pain in, Side pain, Spermatic cords-neuralgia of, Spleen-affections of, Tumours, Urine-disorders of, Vaginismus.

V. Symptoms-General (Nash-310-11)

1. Bruised pain with numbness, stiffness, and lameness in region of Kidney, < in Bed in the morning.
2. Soreness in the region of kidneys, bubbling sensation, < stepping or jarring motion.
3. Rheumatism or gouty pains in the joints, the pains radiate from a centre.

VI. Symptoms-Particular (Nash-310-11)

1. Backache-worse when setting or lying, esp. lying in bed in morning.
2. Rise from a seat with difficulty.
3. Suffering in back aggravated by fatigue as in Rhus t. but, in Berb. v. they are in connection with kidney or urinary troubles.
4. Pains sometimes extend to hips, into bladder and urethra, and the urine itself is changed—turbid, flocculent, clay like, copious, mucous sediment or a reddish or mealy sediment or blood red, but the persistent pains in the back are the leading symptoms.
5. Bubbling sensation in region of kidneys.
6. Sensation of soreness in region of kidneys when jumping down or stepping hard or from any jarring movement.

BISMUTH

I. Introduction (Cow-144)

Synonym: Sub-mitrate of Bismuth.
Preparation: Trituration.

Hahnemann proved it homoeopathically (105 symptom in MMP Vol. I-IInd Ed.).

II. General Analysis (Cow.)

Its chief action is upon the alimentary canal causing irritation and catarrhal inflammation.

III. Suited to (Allen-64)

Person to whom solitude is unbearable, child holds to his mother's hand for company (Kali c., Lil. t., Lyc.), Headache returns every winter. Vomiting of water as soon as it reaches stomach, food retained longer.

IV. Clinical (Clarke-I-287)

Abdominal operations—vomiting after, Angina pectoris, Cholera, Cough, Cystitis, Delirium tremens, Diaphragmitis, Diarrhoea, Gangrene, Gastralgia, Gastritis, Headache, Phlegmasia alba dolens, Stomach-cancer of, Stomatitis, Toothache, Vomiting.

V. Symptoms-General (Nash-368)

1. Diarrhoea; stools watery, profuse, painless and offensive or cadaverously smelling.
2. Vomiting of large quantities and intense thirst; water is vomited the moment it reaches the stomach; food is retained a little longer.
3. Restlessness, anguish, great prostration; pale with sweat, with blue rings around eyes, surface covered with sweat but it is warm sweat.

VI. **Symptoms-Particular** (Nash-368-9)

1. One of the best for Cholera Infantum, where it is sudden in onset and rapid in its course. (Bism., Verat., Kreas.).
2. Stools-watery, profuse, very offensive. Vomiting profuse, of water as soon as taken. Food retained for a while.

   Ars.-Food and water both are vomited. Stool's scanty (Allen 50).
3. Prostration

   Ars. -cold clammy perspiration (Allen 51).

   Verat.-coldness general, with cold sweat.

   Bism. -body is warm and covered with warm sweat. Face deathly pale with blue ring around eyes.
4. Purely Nervous Gastralgia with pain of pressing nature, between shoulders or much burning in stomach (Ars.).
5. Vomiting of enormous quantities of food that seems to have lain in stomach for days.

BORAX

I. Introduction (Cow.-146)

Synonym: Biborate of soda.
Preparation: Either Trituration of the pure Borax or dilutions from a solution composed of one part to 99 of distilled water.

The medicine was first proved by Schreter of Hungary (Chronic Diseases, Vol. I, IInd ed.).

II. General Analysis (Cow.)

Has an important action upon mucous membranes, on which it produces aphthous ulceration (Merc. c.), esp. mouth, intestines, uterus and vagina. Most prominent mental expression is "fear of downward motion".

III. Suited to (Allen-64)

Great anxiety from downward motion in almost all complaints. Children awake suddenly, screaming and grasping cradle, without apparent cause (Apis., Cina., Stram.). Excessive nervousness-easily frightened by slight or sudden sharp sound. (Asar., Calad.).

IV. Clinical (Clarke-I-294)

Aphthae, Corns, Dentition, Diarrhoea, Ear-discharge from, Entropion, Erysipelas, Eye affections, Finger joints-ulcers on, Herpes, Menstruation-painful (membranous), Nipple sore, Nose affections, Pleurisy, Plica polonica, Psoriasis, Screaming, Sea-sickness, Sterility, Syphilitic sore-throat, Taste disordered, Trichiasis, Ulcer, Urine-strong smelling, Vertigo, Zoster.

V. **Symptoms-General** (Nash-412)

1. Dread of downward motion; child jumps and cringes, cries when laying him down, very sensitive to noises.
2. Aphthous sore mouth: greenish stools day and night, mouth very hot.
3. Pain in right pectoral region. Cough with offensive herby tasting expectoration.

VI. **Symptoms-Particular** (Nash 412-14)

1. Great sensitiveness to noise (cough, a sneeze, rustling of news paper a distant shot etc.).
   Bor. ++
   Bell. +
2. Fear of falling from downward motion.
   Bor.-
   Gels.-(Nash noticed this symptom only in intermittent fever).
   Sanic.-
   (During sleep child starts and clings to nurse in Apis., Bell., Cina., Stram.).
3. Aphthous (sore) ulcers in mouth.
4. Eyelashes stick together become gummy and or turn inward.
5. Ears discharge.
6. Stools-greenish day and night. Dry crust in nose, reformed if removed.
7. Leucorrhoea-white, starchy like warm water running down-profuse, thin.
8. Child cries before urinating (If with deposits of sand then Lyc., Sarsa.).
9. For symptoms reported from way back, choice to be made from:—
   Merc. c.,
   Hydras.,
   Sul.,
   Sul. ac.
10. Slight injury, has ulceration of skin, suppurates
    Cham.,
    Hep. s.,

Sil.,
Bor.

11. Pain in right pectoral region; cough with expectoration of an offensive, herby taste.

VII. Black Letter Symptoms (Tyler-135-6)

- The child becomes anxious when dancing; if one rocks it in arms it has an anxious expression of face during downward motion.
- Anxious feeling during downward motion or rocking. Dread of downward motion.
- Very anxious when riding rapidly down hill, contrary to his custom he feels as though it would take away his breath.
- Anxious feeling during downward motion or rocking. (Diarrhoea).
- Vertigo and fullness in head on descending mountain or stairs.
- Aphthae with salivation.
- Aphthae in mouth, on tongue, and inner surface of check, bleeding easily; with great heat and dryness of mouth; with cracked tongue.
- Mouth of infant very hot.
- Aphthae are so tender that they prevent child from nursing.
- Soft, light yellow, mucous stool.
- Worse before urination.
- Frequently cries and screams before the urine passes.
- White albuminous, or starchy Leucorrhoea.
- Leucorrhoea like the white of an egg, with sensation as if warm water were flowing down.
- Acrid Leucorrhoea, appearing for two weeks, between Catamenia, with swelling of labia and inflamed and discharging Duvernis glands.
- Sensation of warm water running down thighs.
- Pleuritic pain in right pectoral region; patient cannot move or breathe without a stitch.
- With every cough and deep inspiration, stiches in the chest.

- Children may be sleeping quietly, and awake suddenly, screaming and holding on to sides of cradle without any apparent cause for so doing.
- The infant frequently cries out in its sleep, and anxiously grasps its mother, as it had been frightened by a dream.
- She cannot fall asleep again for two hours, on account of heat in the whole body, especially in the head.
- Period of dentition and infancy.

BROMIUM

I. Introduction (Cow-151)

Common Name: Bromine, An elementary substance. Preparation: Dilution made from a solution of one part of Bromium to 99 parts of distilled water. 2nd-4th dilution with distilled water, 6th onward with alcohol.

First proved by others, but most of its knowledge is due to Dr. Herring and his provers (Pierce-319).

II. General Analysis (Cow.)

Acts powerfully as irritant upon mucous membranes esp. of respiratory tract and larynx; Membranous Croup and Diphtheria. It produces violent Gastritis, depression and collapse. Intense inflammation in respiratory tract causes membranous croup and diphtheria.

III. Suited to (Allen-67)

Person with light blue eyes, flaxen hair, light eye brows, fair, delicate skin, red, checked, scrofulous girls, sensation of cobweb on the face (Baryt. c., Bor., Graph.).

IV. Clinical (Clarke-I-305)

Apoplexy, Asthma, Breast-cancer of, Breast-tumour of, Cancer, Cough, Croup, Diphtheria, Dysmenorrhoea, Emphysema, Feet-pain in, Fistula lachrymalis, Glands enlarged, Goitre, Heart-disease of; hypertrophy of, Laryngismus, Migraine, Parotid gland-induration of, Respiration-affections of, Scrofula, Seaside-effects of, Testicles-induration of, Throat sore, Tonsil-enlarged; inflamed, Trachea-irritation in, Tuberculosis, Ulcer, Uterus-air in, Vagina-air in, Vertigo

V. Symptoms-Particular (Nash-356)

1. An important medicine in laryngeal affection
2. Glandular affections

Carb. a. Con.	pains lancinating cutting or burning	glands stony hard with a cancerous tendency.
Brom.	-Pain not characteristic	

3. Diphtheria
   Brom.-membrane first forms in the bronchi, trachea, or larynx, running upwards.
   Lyc. -Just opposite of Brom., often forms in nose and often runs downward.
4. Croup with rattle of mucous but no expectoration.
   Hep. s.,
   Brom.
5. Great danger of suffocation from accumulation of mucous.
   Ant. tar.-in Bronchi.
   Brom.-in Larynx.
6. Sensation of cobwebs on face.
   Baryt. c.,
   Bor.,
   Graph.,
   Brom.
7. Fan like motion of alae nasi.
   Ant. tar.,
   Lyc.
8. Hypertrophy of heart
   Caust.-from gymnastics.
   Lac can.-Membranous dysmenorrhoea.

VI. Black Letter Symptoms (Tyler-141-42)

- She does not feel, as she generally does, but can't tell why.
- Parotids, mostly left, affected.
- Swelling and hardness of left parotid, warm to touch.
- Suppuration of left parotid: discharge watery and excoriating: swelling remains hard and unyielding. (Especially after scarlet fever).

- Long-continued obstinate Coryza with soreness beneath nose and on margin of nose.
- Grey, earthy colour of Face.
- Stony hard swelling of Glands, especially on lower jaw and throat. Diphtheria or croup.
- Periodically much pain in left hypochondrium and iliac regions.
- Pain violent, as if a sore inside.
- Black Faecal Stools.
- Varices, anus, worse application of cold or warm water.
- Loud emission of flatus from vagina.
- Cold sensation in Larynx, with cold feeling on inspiring.
- Chronic hoarseness: loss of voice: he can't speak clearly.
- Scraping and rawness provoking dry cough; in the evening.
- A feeling as if the pit of the throat were pressed against the trachea.
- Cough with paroxysms of suffocation.
- Rattling of mucus in larynx when coughing: cough sounds croupy.
- Diphtheria, when disease commences in larynx, and comes up to fauces, or in some cases where it runs down to Larynx, with croupy cough and rattling of mucus.
- No choking with cough, as with Hep. s.
- Much rattling in larynx when breathing: more when coughing.
- Danger of suffocation from phlegm in larynx. (Ant. tar. has rattling lower down in chest.)
- Croupous inflammation formed by exuberant growth of fungi (Diphtheria).
- Constriction of chest; no cough; with difficulty of breathing.
- Asthma of sailors as soon as they go ashore.
- Symptoms of croup during whooping cough.
- Icy cold forearms.

BRYONIA ALBA

I. Introduction (Cow-154)

Synonym: Bryonia Alba.
Natural Order: Cucurbitaceae.
Common Name: White Bryony.
Habitat: High climbing perennial plant growing in hedges, esp. in Germany and France.
Preparation: Tincture from fresh root.

The medicine was proved by Hahnemann and his fellow provers. Total symptoms 780 (MMP Vol. I-3rd Ed).

II. General Analysis (Cow.)

It acts especially and powerfully upon serous membranes and their viscera, lungs, brain and liver, then synovial membranes of respiratory and alimentary tracts. Conditions produced are between inflammations, where effusions, exudations or infiltrations are about to occur. Its chief expressions are—stitching pains, tearing pains, worse by motion.

III. Suited to (Allen-68)

Irritable, vehement and angry, dark complexioned, firm muscle fibre, dry, nervous, slender (Nux. v.). Best suited to gouty rheumatic diathesis. Constant motion of left arm and leg. Headache from constipation (Aloe., Collin., Op.); Constipation at sea (Plat.). Fever-bone pain, lies quietly. Complaints-when warm weather sets in after cold days, cold ice in hot weather, chilling when over heated. < motion > Rest, lying on painful side.

IV. Clinical (Clarke-I-310)

Alcoholism, Amenorrhoea, Anger-effects of, Aphthae, Apoplexy, Asthma, Bilious attack, Brain-affections of, Breast inflamed, Bronchitis, Cancer, Chill-effects of, Chlorosis, Constipation, Consumption, Coryza, Cough, Dentition, Diaphragm-rheumatism of, Diarrhoea, Dropsy, Dyspepsia, Eczema, Enteric fever, Eruptions, Gastroenteritis, Haemorrhage, Hands swollen, Headache, Heart-inflammation of, Hernia, Hiccough, Hydrocele, Hydrocephalus, Influenza, Intermittent fever, Jaundice, Joints-pain in, Lactation disordered, Liver disorder, Lumbago, Measles, Meningitis, Menstruation-vicarious, Miliaria, Milk fever, Myalgia, Nephritis, Nose-bleed, Peritonitis, Phlegmasia alba dolens, Pleurisy, Pleurodynia, Pneumonia, Pregnancy-morning cough of; sickness of, Puerperal fever, Pyuria, Relapsing fever, Remittent fever, Rheumatism, Scarlatina, Screaming, Side-pain in, Sleep-anxious dreams in, Spina bifida, Stiff-neck, Suppressed eruptions-effects of, Thirst, Tongue coated, Toothache, Trachea-pain in, Vertigo, Waking-starts and screams on, Water-brash, Whooping-cough, Yellow fever.

V. **Symptoms-General** (Nash-29)

1. *All complaints < on motion.*
2. *Dryness* of mucous membranes generally (lips, mouth, stomach, wants drink in large quantities, at long intervals; intestines, dry hard stool as if burnt). Effusions in serous membranes(meninges, pleura, peritoneum, etc.).
3. *Constipation* (no desire) or diarrhoea < mornings on beginning to move.
4. *Stitching pains*, especially in serous membranes and joints.
5. Sitting up causes nausea and faintness.
6. Modalities < from motions, warm weather after cold, > from quiet, lying on painful side.
7. Suitable to dry, spare, nervous, slender persons, of irritable disposition; rheumatic tendency. Complaints in hot weather, or exposure to dry, cold air, in wet weather (Rhus t.).
8. Cough, dry hard, racking, with scanty expectoration; with splitting headache; delirium, about the business

of the day (typhoid) headache < stooping; ironing, hot weather, coughing; motion, vertigo, with nausea, and faintness; < from sitting up after lying down. Pressure, as from a stone at pit of stomach, relieved by eructation.

9. Vicarious menstruation; nose bleeds when menses should appear. (Phos.)
10. Mammae heavy, of a stony hardness; pale but hard; hot and painful.
11. Rheumatism of joints; with pale swelling, great pain, worse on touch or least motion.

VI. Symptoms-Particular (Nash-30-35)

1. *Aggravation from least motion,* suffering of almost any and every kind relieved greatly by lying still, then Bry. is first medicine to be thought of.
2. Better from Pressure.
   Lies on painful part-Reverse of Bell., Kali c.
   - (a) *Motion of affected part worse.*
     Dulc.,
     Ferr.,
     Puls.,
     Rhus t.,
     Sul.
   - (b) *Excessive Dryness of Mucous surfaces* (from lips to anus).
     - (i) *Excessive thirst.*
       -Ars. (small quantity of water at short intervel).
       -Bry. (large quantity at long intervals-a little does not satisfy).
     - (ii) Stools hard, dry as if burnt.
3. *Hard dry cough with little or no expectoration with pain in chest-Bry.*
   Nat. s.-loose cough with soreness.
4. Serous membrane affections (Lining of a cavity which has no direct external air lining of large cavities on a bdominal).
   - (i) Ist stage Inflammation-Acon.
     IInd stage of inflammation after the stage of serous affections has set in

Bell.,
Ferr. phos.

(ii) *With stitching pain* < night, motion. Cries out sharply with pain.
Bry.-on motion
Kali bich.-any time

(iii) Stitching pain of the serous membrane.
Bry.-> pressure < motion
Kali c.-No effect of pressure
Nat. m.
Squil. } stitching pains.
Merc. v.
Apis.-cries out with stinging pain

(Sul. precedes and follows all these three great remedies [Bry., Kali c., Apis.] for affections of serous cavities)

5. *Indigestion*

(a) sensation of stone in the stomach.
Bry.-thirst, Nausea < Motion
Nux. v.-little or no thirst-sour Nausea in AM and after eating.
Puls.-Thirst nil-nausea in evening and after eating.

(b) *gastric disorder.*
Bry.-Dietic error esp. when warm weather sets in after cold.
Nux. v.-Continued over eating, abuse of drugs, coffee, tobacco etc.
Puls.-Too rich food, fats, ice cream (in excess).

(c) Diarrhoea.
Bry.-morning, < movement, over eating, in heat of summer.
Nux. v.-morning, over-eating, dysenteric type.

Puls.-night, great rumbling.

6. Bursting headache < stooping < coughing < hot weather.
7. Menses alters with epistaxis-Phos. (Allen-69)
8. Mastitis (breast sore, hot, hard, pain-must support breast-Phyt. (Allen)

9. Desire to take long breath-must expand the lungs.
   Bry., Cact.., Ign., Nat. s.
10. Cough < coming from open air to warm room (Nat. c.) < Moving
11. Cough hurts, holds chest with hands.
    Bry.,
    Eup. perf.,
    Nat. s.
12. Suppression of milk, menses, measles or rash of Scarlatina.

VII. Black Letter Symptoms

(Tyler-147-150)

- ANXIETY; he is apprehensive about the future.
- Irrational talking about his business.
- Very ill humoured; troubled with needless anxiety.
- Morose: everything puts him out of humour.
- Dreams full of quarrelling and vexatious things.
- Dreams all night very vividly of anxious and careful attention to his business. In his dreams he is occupied with household affairs.
- During sleep was continually busy with what he read the evening previous.
- Delirious prattling about business to be attended to.
- Confusion of the head.
- Vertigo as soon as he rises from his chair.
- On rising from bed in morning, dizzy and whirling, as if head were turning in a circle.
- Headache commences in the morning,when first opening and moving eyes.
- Pressive frontal headache, very much increased by stooping.
- In the occiput, obtuse pain.
- A pressing pain in the occiput, with drawing down into the neck; relieved towards noon.
- Digging pressure in the front of the brain, with pressing towards the forehead, especially violent when stooping or walking quickly. A walk tires him very much.

- Headache on stooping, as if everything would fall out at the forehead; as if everything would press out at the forehead.
- Pressive pain above the right eye, followed by dull pressing pain in the occiput, whence it spread over the whole body, and continued more or less severe the whole day; on quick motion and after eating the pain became so severe that it seemed like a distinct pulsation within the head.
- An out-pressing pain in both temples.
- Pain in left eyeball, especially violent on moving the ball.
- Frequent lachrymation.
- In the morning eyes as if gummed up with matter.
- Nosebleed for a quarter of an hour in the morning.
- Red, hot, soft puffiness of the face.
- Drawing, sometimes twitching toothache in the molars of left upper jaw, only during and after eating, at the same time the teeth felt too long and as if they waggled to and fro.
- Pain as if a tooth were screwed in and then pulled out, momentarily relived by cold water.
- Toothache about 3 AM which becomes aggravated on lying on the painful side, and then goes away if one lies on the painful cheek.
- Very white, coated tongue. Tongue thickly coated white.
- Dryness in the mouth: mouth very dry. Violent thirst.
- Collection of much soapy, frothy saliva in the mouth.
- Insipid, sticky taste in the mouth: he has almost no taste.
- Offensive, bitter taste. Intensely bitter taste and the inclination to vomit.
- Frequent drinking of cold water relieved bitter taste & inclination to vomit.
- Excessive thirst.
- Great thirst, obliged to drink much cold water.
- Great thirst: she can and must drink a great deal at once.

- Excessive hunger.
- No appetite for milk, but when he takes it the appetite for it comes, and he commences to relish it.
- Great longing for coffee.
- After a meal, bitter Eructation: or sourish.
- After eating, pressure in stomach as if a stone lay there & made him cross.
- As if a stone lay in stomach, after eating ; epigastric region painful to touch: painful to pressure. (only here is Bryonia not releived by pressure, i.e., in stomach and abdomen.
- Pasty offensive evacuations in the afternoon followed by burning in anus.
- Diarrhoea preceded by cutting in the stomach.
- Obstinate constipation.
- Dry, parched stool, with effort.
- Urine dark, almost brown.
- Fluent coryza for eight days.
- Severe coryza without cough.
- Viscid phlegm in the fauces that was detached by hawking.
- Dry cough.
- Irritation to hacking cough: it seems as if some mucous were in the wind pipe; when he coughs for some time he feels a pain there compounded of soreness and pressure: the pain becomes more violent by speaking and smoking tobacco.
- When he comes from the open into a warm room he has a feeling as if a vapour were in the windpipe, which compels him to cough. He feels as if he could not breathe in enough air.
- Viscid phlegm in the windpipe, detached by frequent hacking cough.
- When coughing it always goes into the head like a pressure.
- Stitches in sternum on coughing he was obliged to hold chest with hand.
- Internal heat in the chest.
- Sharp outward shooting pain under the right nipple, in the cavity of the chest, only on expiring.

CACTUS GRANDIFLORUS

I. Introduction (Cow-164)

Synonym: Cactus Grandiflorous.
Natural Order: Cactaceae.
Common Name: Night blooming Cereus.
Habitat: A flowering plant native of Mexico and West Indies.
Preparation: Tincture from the fresh flowers and youngest twigs.

II. General Analysis (Cow.)

Acts mainly upon the heart and arteries causing irritability, hyper aesthesia, neuralgia, spasm and palpitation of the heart. It acts upon the heart, lungs, stomach causing indigestion and excessive acidity in the latter, and asthma and contraction in the lungs. Intermittent fever with regular periodicity (Cedr.). *Chief characteristic-constrictive sensation in various part of the body, esp. in the region of the heart as if bound with an iron hoop.*

III. Suited to (Allen-71)

Sanguinic congestions of people of plethoric habit (Acon.) often resulting in Haemorrhage-Fear of death; believes the disease incurable (Ars.). Constriction-feels whole body caged tight. Sanguinous apoplexy (stroke, unconsciousness sudden).

IV. Clinical (Clark-I-323)

Aneurism, Angina pectoris, Apoplexy, Arteries- atheroma of, Asthma, Bladder-paralysis of, Brain-congestion of, Bronchitis, Diaphragm-rheumatism of, Dropsy, Ear-inflammation of, Fistula, Goitre-exophthalmic, Haematuria, Haemorrhage, Headache, Heart-affections of; hypertrophy of, Indigestion, Intermittent fever, Lungs-haemorrhage from,

Melancholy, Menstruation painful, Miliaria, Neuralgia, Otitis, Ovaritis, Pneumonia, Prostate-affections of, Rheumatism, Sun-effects of, Sunstroke, Traumatic fever, Vaginismus.

V. Symptoms-General (Nash-224)

1. *Constriction of the heart*, as if an iron band prevented its normal movement < lying on left side.
2. Constriction, general; of heart, chest, bladder, rectum, uterus, vagina,etc.
3. *Haemorrhage* in connection with heart troubles; nose, lungs, stomach, rectum, bladder.
4. *Palpitation*; day or night; worse when walking and lying on left side; approach of menses.
5. *Fear of death*; believes the disease incurable.

VI. Symptoms-Particular (Nash-224)

1. *Great heart remedy* (Dig.).
   Sensation of constriction of heart as if an iron band prevented its normal movement.
   Iod.-Sensation as if heart was squeezed together.
   Lil. t.-as if grasped and released alternately.
   Lach.-Constriction on awakening-throws off covering.
   Ars.-Constriction or obstruction on walking.
2. *Sensation of constriction* is found in other parts such as chest, bladder, rectum, uterus, vagina, etc.
   Constriction is general characteristic of this medicine.
3. *Heart troubles* caused quite aptly by inflammatory rheumatism.
4. *Symptoms found with heart troubles*:
   (i) heavy pain on vertex like a weight (Glon., Lach. at climacteric.).
   (ii) any haematuria or Haemorrhage from nose, haematemasis, bleeding from anus,seeming to be in sympathy with heart trouble indicates Cact.
5. *Valuable heart and chest symptoms*:
   -Oppression of chest or difficult breathing-chest cannot be expanded.

-Periodical attacks of suffocation with fainting, cold sweat on face, loss of pulse.
-Fluttering or palpitation of heart < when walking or lying on left side.
-Irregularity of heart action, intermittent pulse, valvular murmurs in organic diseases of heart.
-Palpitation < on left side (Nat. m.).
-Oedema of left hand, foot or leg.
-Rheumatism of all joints beginning in upper extremities (Ledum.-lower).
-Numbness of left arm-Acon., aching-Rhus t.

CALCAREA CARBONICA

I. Introduction (Cow-169)

Synonym: Calcarea Ostrearum Hahnemaniani.
Preparation: Trituration of the pure white middle layer of the oyster shell.

It was first proved by Hahnemann who recorded 1630 symptoms in his "Chronic Diseases" (Vol. I-P) (Pierce-pg. 329).

II. General Analysis

Tyler gives five definite uses of this drug-teething, rickets, anaemia, tuberculosis, mental deficiency and decay. It acts primaryly upon vegetative systems, affecting all organs and systems of the body including composition of blood. In affecting the processes of assimilation, Calc. c. resembles in its effect upon three great disorders of nutrition-scrofula, tuberculosis, and rachites which are its chief sphere of usefulness.

III. Suited to (Allen-73)

Light complexion and leucophlegmatic, blond hair, fair skinned, tendency to grow fat in youth. Pale, weak, timid, easily tired when walking. Girls fleshy plethoric, grow too rapidly. Menses too early, too profuse, too long-lasting. The least exertion causes menses (Sul., Tuberc.). Children with red face, flabby muscles, sweat easily and take cold easily in consequence.

IV. Clinical (Clarke-I-338)

Abdomen-large, Acidity, Alcohol-effects of, Anaemia, Ankles weak, Appetite depraved, Beard-sycosis of, Bone disease, Brachial neuralgia, Breasts painful, Bronchial glands-affections of, Calculi, Caries, Cataract, Chilblains, Chorea, Colds, Constipation, Corpulency, Coryza, Cough, Coxalgia,

Croup, Crusta lactea, Debility, Delirium tremens, Dentition, Diabetes, Diarrhoea, Dropsy, Dyspepsia, Ear affections, Epilepsy, Epulis, Eye affections, Fever-intermittent, Fistula, Gall-stones, Glandular swellings, Gleet, Goitre, Gonorrhoea, Gouty swellings, Headache, Hernia, Herpes, Hydrocephalus, Hypochondriasis, Hysteria, Impotence, Joint affections, Lactation defective, Leukocythemia, Leucorrhoea, Lupus, Masturbation, Melancholia, Menstruation disordered, Milk fever, Miller's phthisis, Miscarriage, Molluscum contagiosum, Naevus, Nervous fever, Neuralgia, Night-terrors, Paralysis, Parotitis, Peritonitis, Perspiration, Plethora, Polypi, Pregnancy, Prosopoplagia, Psoriasis palmaris, Ranula, Renal colic, Rhagades, Rheumatism, Rickets, Ringworm, Sciatica, Scrofula, Skin-affections of, Sleep disordered, Sleeplessness, Smell disordered, Spinal affections, Stone-cutter's phthisis, Strains, Sycosis, Sycosis menti, Tabes mesenterica, Tape-worm, Taste disordered, Teeth carious, Toothache, Trachea-affections of, Tuberculosis, Tumours, Typhoid, Urticaria, Uterine affections, Varices, Vertigo, Walking late, Warts, Whitlow, Worms.

V. Symptoms-General (Nash-71)

1. Deficient or irregular bone development. (fontanelle open, crooked spine, deformed extremities).
2. Leucophlegmatic temperament.
3. Fair, fat, flabby, obesic.
4. Coldness, general and local, subjective and objective, especially as if had on cold, damp stockings. Affections from working in cold water.
5. Sweats general (night sweats and on exertion). Local, head (children) axillae, hands, feet, etc.
6. Digestive tract sour-(sour taste, eructation, vomiting sour curds, diarrhoea).
7. Great debility; can't walk far or go upstairs for short breath; easily strained.
8. Modalities; < cold air, ascending, or exertion; straining from lifting.

VI. Symptoms-Particular (Nash 72-77)

1. Constitutional remedy-may come in use in almost any form of disease.
2. Temperament is leucophlegmatic.
3. Patients (esp. children and young people) are constitutionally fat or inclined to obesity (Graph.), colour of skin is white or chalky pale, torpid disposition, sluggish or slow in movements.

   Constitutional Trio-Calc. c., Sul., Lyc.

   Obesity of Calc. c. and eruptive tendency of Sul.-combined effect covers-Hep. s.).
4. Malnutrition.
5. Bones-tardy development of bone tissue with lymphatic enlargements.

   -curvature of bones, esp. long such as spine.

   -extremely deformed, crooked.

   -softening of the bones, fontanelles remain open too long, with profuse sweat on head of large-headed children.
6. Nutrition impaired with tendency to glandular enlargements.
7. Granular, vegetatious, polypi (in nose, ear, bladder, uterus etc.).
8. Coldness-Cold, damp feet, sensation of cold damp stockings as if, coldness of legs with night sweats, internal and external sensation of cold in various parts of head, with pale puffed face, inward coldness, aversion to open air, the least cold air goes right through, sensation of coldness in single parts or general-Calc. c. (Cistus., Helod.).
9. Night sweats with debilitating diseases. In all sweating of Cal. surface is generally cold.
10. Digestive tract-sour-sour vomiting, sour diarrhoea, sour smell of whole body (offensive-Sul.). Longing for eggs. Stomach distended like an inverted saucer, while body is emaciated. Diarrhoea < afternoon. > constipated.
11. Skin-Eczema capites or milk crusts.

    -cold, soft and flabby.

12. Respiratory organs-one of the best remedies for pulmonary consumption.
    Middle and upper portion of right lung (Sul.-upper left).
13. Chest painfully sensitive to touch and inspiration.
14. Painless hoarseness < morning.
15. Shortness of breath on walking, esp. on ascending.
16. Women-too early and profuse in menses; who have habitually cold feet to knees.
17. Tendency to looseness of the bowels < afternoon.
18. Appetite failing and emaciation progressing.

VII. Black Letter Symptoms

(Tyler-158-164)

- Thinking is difficult.
- Visions of faces and persons, when eyes are closed.
- Fears that she will lose her reason or that people will observe her confusion of mind.
- Anxiety-shuddering and dread as soon as evening comes on, with fear of death.
- Great anxiety, restlessness and palpitation.
- Despairing, hopeless of ever getting well, with fear of death; tormenting all around, day and night.
- Children self willed, inclined to grow fat.
- After exerting mind; hyperaemia of head; chorea; trembling spells.
- Excitement brings on dysmenorrhea; least excitement endangers return of catamenia, or causes.
- Vertigo; when climbing to high places; on going upstairs, or up a hill; on suddenly raising or turning head, even when at rest; on walking in open air, as if he would tumble, especially on suddenly turning HEAD; with stupefaction and a sensation of falling (neurosis cordis) with inclination to fall backward or sideways; with headache; nausea and vomiting, incarcerated flatulence; accompanied by nausea and a feeling as though one would fall unconscious; with unsteadiness in thighs when walking rapidly; in Addison's disease; during intervals of epileptic spasms.

- Stupefying pressive pain in forehead, with confusion of senses and dullness of whole head, while reading; he was obliged to stop and did not know where he was.
- Tearing headache above eyes down to nose, with nausea.
- Headache begins in occiput and spreads to top of head, so severe that she thinks head will burst, and that she will go crazy.
- Concussive, stitching, pulsating pains in head, as if it would split, with cough.
- Internal and external sensation of coldness of various parts of head, as if a piece of ice was lying against it, with pale puffed face.
- Congestion of head; with heat and stupefying headache; with red puffed face; with toothache; during night; < in morning when awakening, and from spiritous drinks.
- Chronic hydrocephalus.
- Burning in vertex; also after grief.
- Internal and external sensation of coldness of one (right) side of head, as if a piece of ice was lying there; < weather changing; in early morning; from motion in open air; < on lying down.
- Sweating of head very profuse, rolling down face in large, bead like drops; the pillow is wet for some distance around child's head. Tinea. Chalk-like stools.
- Nocturnal sweats of head.
- Head too large, fontanelles not closing.
- Rachitis.
- Open fontanelles, with large head and with sweating of same; children leuco-phlegmatic, very fat and of leaden weight; abdomen hard and distended with sour-swelling diarrhoea.
- Scratches head impatiently on getting awake or when disturbed in sleep.
- Tinea favosa; thick scabs covered with thick pus.
- Crusta serpiginosa; Herpes circinatus.
- Great photophobia < in evening; agglutination of lids in morning (EYE). Cataract.

- Horrid visions when EYES are closed.
- Dilated pupils; often indicated after Sul.
- Fundus haematodes with opacity of cornea.
- Dimness of cornea; opacity; maculae.
- Pustules on cornea, much lachrymation and excessive photophobia; < by gaslight, or in morning, and in changes of weather.
- Ophthalmia; from taking cold; entrance of foreign body; in the new born; scrofulous; arthritic.
- Inflammation and swelling of outer and inner EAR.
- Otorrhoea muco-purulent, affecting principally right ear; enlarged glands.
- Ulceration, then granulation, then polypi; great stench.
- Nasal polypi, with loss of smell.
- Swelling of NOSE and upper lip, in children.
- Face looks old and wrinkled.
- Face puffed up, in children.
- Lips chapped and cracked; corners of mouth ulcerated.
- Chewing motion of jaws during sleep.
- Painful swelling of sub maxillary GLANDS.
- Hard, painful swelling of sub maxillary glands; painful tension when chewing; sticking pain when touched.
- TEETH can't endure air or any coldness.
- Difficult dentition, with Rachitis. Eclampsia. Cholera Infantum. Hydrocephalus. Crusta Lactea. Infantile catarrh. Laryngo-trachiitis. Bronchitis. Bronchial catarrh. Marasmus. Urticaria. Chorea.
- TONGUE dry, does not like to talk. (Compare Phos. ac. and Bell.).
- Sore THROAT marked; cellular tissue around cervical glands swollen; nose sore; obstructed. Ravenous hunger, with wake STOMACH.
- Appetite poor, with an aversion to meat and a craving for boiled eggs.
- Complete loss of appetite.
- Longing for boiled eggs.
- Aversion to meat.
- Sour vomiting, especially during dentition.

- Vomiting and diarrhoea of teething children.
- Pit of stomach swollen like a saucer turned bottom up; painful to pressure.
- Bloating in region of stomach, compelling him to undo his clothing.
- Tight clothes about hypochondria are unbearable.
- Pains more on left side, especially under left hypochondrium; tearing stitching pains in left chest to hypochondrium.
- Flatulence with gurgling in right side of ABDOMEN.
- Abdomen much distended; hard.
- Mesenteric glands hard and swollen in children; abdomen feels as if filled with stones or ovoid bodies.
- Mesenteric atrophy.
- Emaciated everywhere, except abdomen.
- Soreness of naval; a moist excrescence like proud flesh from navel of infants. (Kali c., Nat. m.).
- Diarrhoea of sour smell.
- Watery stools.
- Tapeworm and ascarides with stool.
- Tapeworm; after Graph.
- Polypi and varices of Bladder.
- Increases Sexuality and provokes emissions, but unusual weakness follows indulgence and ejaculation is tardy.
- Impotence.
- Consequences of onanism or of too frequent coitus; pressing pain in hand and back; lassitude and weakness in lower limbs; knees seem to give way; sweats easily; debility; hands tremble.
- Frequent nocturnal involuntary emissions.
- Itching and burning of genitals of both sexes.
- Menses will not appear; in plethora.
- Menses; too early; last too long; too profuse.
- The least excitement brings on a return of profuse catamenia.
- Metrorrhagia.
- Leucorrhoea; like milk with itching and burning. Before or after menses; during micturation; profuse at times; in fits and starts; worse after exercise; with

great debility; with stinging in os and aching in vagina; with burning in cervical canal; with accumulation of mucus between labia and thighs; with chlorosis; in scrofulous women.

- Leucorrhoea with pruritus; white, milky but not thick; heat of parts.
- Leucorrhoea thick, yellow; by day, when urinating.
- Frequent leucorrhoea between menses, which are too early and profuse.
- Vaginal polypi and fistula.
- Clumsy, awkward, easily falls; tired from short walk, from a general feeling of lameness in pelvis. Cramp in toes, or soles of feet, during pregnancy.
- False labour pains, running upward.
- Excessive lactation; also hectic and sweat; debility as a consequence.
- Breasts distended, milk scanty; she is cold; feels cold air very readily; there is a want of vitality to secrete milk.
- Deficient milk; mammae not swollen.
- Breasts hard, but not red.
- Milk disagrees with infant.
- Crusts on head in nursing children.
- Inflammation of eyes with new-born children.
- Difficult teething of children.
- Painless hoarseness; could scarcely speak; < in morning.
- Hoarse, hardly audible voice.
- Loud breathing through nose.
- Shortness of breath after walking and on going up slightest ascent.
- Mucus rattles in chest on expiration; < when lying and in evening.
- Night cough.
- Cough < in morning on rising and in early evening.
- Acts upon upper and middle portion of right lung.
- Sore pains in chest, as if beaten; < during inspiration.
- Secretion of milk too abundant; galactorrhea.
- Tuberculous consumption.

- Chest painfully sensitive to touch, and on inspiration.
- Cervical glands swollen.
- Glands of neck swollen, with eruption on head.
- Easily overstrains himself from lifting, from which neck becomes stiff and rigid, with headache.
- Pressure between and under shoulder blades.
- Weakness and trembling in legs, especially above and below knees.
- Swelling of knees.
- Cold, damp feet.
- Sensation in feet and legs as if she had on cold deep stockings.
- Child is very Backward in learning to walk; seems to forget how to walk.
- Epilepsy; Before the attack sense of something running in arms, or from pit of stomach down through abdomen into feet; sudden attacks of vertigo; loss of consciousness without Convulsion; pharyngeal spasms, followed by desire to swallow. Causes; vexation, fright; onanism; protracted, intermittent; suppression of chronic eruption. Worse at night, during solstice and full moon, with howling and shouting.
- Great weakness.
- Easy relapses, one does not continue to convalesce.
- Great loss of power on walking, esp. in limbs, with exhausting sweat.
- She was unable to go upstairs, and became very much exhausted from it.
- The same disagreeable idea always rouses the sick as often as they fall into a light slumber.
- When closing eyes, horrid visions.
- Child chews and swallows in sleep.
- Hectic Fever ; with alternate chills and heat; frequent attacks of flushes of heat, with anguish and palpitation of heart, or constant shuddering in evening, with red cheeks; skin dry, withered; sweats easily; great debility; after prolonged or profuse lactation, loss of fluids, tuberculosis, etc.

- Partial sweats; nape of neck; chest; hands.
- Intermittent fever after abuse of quinine; chronic forms with scrofula; chill commences in stomach, agonizing weight, increasing with chill and disappearing with it; with people who work much in cold water; cachectic constitutions; suppressed Eruption; desire for eggs.
- Typhoid fever, during aggravation which precedes rash (14th day), palpitation, tremulous pulse, anxiety, red face, delirium, jerks; short, hacking cough; excessive diarrhoea.
- Morning sweat.
- Cold feet at night in bed.
- Aversion to open air; the least cold goes right through.
- Worse during full moon.
- Chlorosis.
- Varicose veins; burning in veins.
- Inflammation, painful swelling and induration of gland.
- Cystic swellings.
- Tardy development of Bony Tissues, with lymphatic enlargements.
- Softening of bones ; fontanelles remaining open too long, and skull very large; swelling of joints.
- Curvature of bones, especially of spine and long bones.
- Extremities deformed, crooked (Rachitis).
- Hip disease; second stage; scratches head on awakening; craves boiled eggs, swollen glands; diarrhoea, etc.
- Muscles soft and flabby.
- Nutrition impaired, with tendency to glandular engorgement.
- Chaps, or rhagades, especially in those who work in water.
- Eczema, thin, moist scabs upon head, with swollen cervical glands; eczema behind ears. (Graph.).
- Diseases of children, especially during Dentition.
- Leuco-phlegmatic temperament in childhood.

- Constitution. Children; self-willed; fair, plumb; Fat, flabby, with red face, sweat easily, and readily take cold; large head and abdomens open fontanelles and sutures, and crooked legs.
- The young who grow too fat and heavy.
- During dentition. Eclampsia.
- Nervous, haemorrhoidal, plethoric and lymphatic constitutions; disposed to grow fat.
- Leuco-phlegmatic; light complexion, blue eyes, blonde hair, fair, skin.
- Compatible ; before Lyc., Nux. v., Phos., Plat., Sil.; after Cham., Nit. ac., Nux. v., Puls., Sul. (especially if pupils dilate).
- Incompatible; before Nit. ac. and Sul., according to Hahnemann.

CALCAREA PHOSPHORICA

I. Introduction (Cow-177)

Common Name: Phosphate of Lime.
Preparation: Triturations of the precipitation of phosphate of lime.

This medicine was first proved by Dr. Hering about 1837 (Pierce-336).

II. General Analysis (Cow.)

Affects exclusively the vegetative system, causing defective nutrition imperfect cell development, and consequent decay of tissue esp. in osseous and glandular system. (This medicine was "adopted by" Shuesslar as one of his 12 tissues.)

III. Suited to (Allen-76)

Anaemic and dark complexioned persons, thin instead of fat. During 1st and IInd dentition of scrofulous child. Oozing of bloody fluid from navel of child (Urine-Hyo.). Fontanelles and sutures remain open too long.

IV. Clinical (Clarke I-358)

Anaemia, Ankles weak, Back-weakness of, Bone affections, Brain-fag, Bright's disease, Cholera infantum, Chorea, Consumption, Cretinism, Debility, Dentition, Diabetes, Dyspepsia, Emissions, Enuresis, Epilepsy, Erotomania, Face-boils on, Fistula, Fracture, Gleet, Gonorrhoea, Headaches, Hernia, Hydrocele, Hygroma, Joint affections, Leucorrhoea, Lumbago, Nymphomania, Phosphaturia, Rheumatism, Rickets, Self-abuse, Spermatorrhoea, Spina bifida, Stiff-neck, Strabismus, Testicles swollen, Throat sore, Tobacco-habit, Tonsil enlarged, Uterus-prolapse of; polypi of, Yawning.

V. Symptoms-General (Nash-77)

1. Tardy closing or re-opening of fontanelles in slim, emaciated children with sweaty heads.
2. Diarrhoea with entero-colitis, stool passes with much flatulence and spluttering noise.
3. Rheumatic troubles < in fall or spring, when air is full of melting snow.

VI. Symptoms-Particular (Nash-77)

1. Over tardy bone development, it is best suited to spare subjects. Sweaty head is also more prominent in Calc. phos. than Sil.
2. Wants to eat.
   Calc. phos.-hamrind, indigestable things (Mag. c.– Meat scrofulous child in).
   Calc. c.-Egg.
3. Diarrhoea-Splitting loud noise with green stool at the time of passing. Best suited to shrunken, emaciated, and very anaemic child (Marasmus).
4. Rheumatic troubles < spring and fall when the air is cold and damp.
5. Broken Bones , when they refuse to knit.
   { Calc. phos., Symp.- } (Best Combination)
6. Headache of school girls.
   Calc. phos.-anaemic
   Nat. m.
7. Feels Complaints more when thinks of them.
   Calc. phos.,
   Oxal. ac.,
   Helon. d.
8. Colic at every attempt to eat (Allen).

VII. Black Letter Symptoms (Tyler-166-167)

- She wishes to be at home, and when at home to go out; goes from place to place (compare Ars.).
- Headache of school girls with diarrhoea.

- Sensation in eye as if something in it; renewed if others talk about it.
- Slowness in teething; also in closing of fontanellas; complaints during teething.
- Chronic enlargement of tonsil.
- Relaxed sore throat.
- Craves bacon, harm, salted or smoked meats. Much Flatulence.
- Cholera Infantum.
- At every attempt to eat, bellyache.
- Flabby, sunken abdomen.
- Fistula in ano, alternating with chest symptoms, or in persons who have pain in all the joints from any change of weather.
- Uterine displacements with rheumatic pains.
- After prolonged nursing.
- Chest difficulty associated with fistula in ano.
- Stiffness of neck after drought of air.
- Rheumatism of Joints with cold or numb feeling.
- Weariness on going up stairs.
- Pains with sensations of crawling, numbness, coldness.
- Copious night sweats in Phthisis.
- Chronic Gonorrhoea in anaemic subject.
- Rheumatism pertaining particularly to cold weather, getting well in Spring and returning next Autumn.
- Can't get awake in early morning.
- Anaemia and chlorosis.
- Non-union of fractured bones.
- Acute affections of the lungs.
- Large pedunculated nasal polypi; polypi of rectum and uterus.
- Rachitis; fontanellas wide open; diarrhoea, emaciation.
- Flabby, shrunken, emaciated children.
- Phosphatic diathesis.
- Child refuses the breast; milk has a saltish taste.
- Involuntary sighing.
- Worse cold; change of weather.

- Guernsey; A subject for this remedy does not present so clear and white a complexion as is called for by Calc. c. Patient more of dirty white or brownish colour.

CAMPHORA

I. Introduction (Cow-181)

Synonym: Laurus camphora.
Natural Order: Lauracae.
Common Name: Camphor.
Habitat-Its tree is found in Central China, Japanese islands and Formosa.
Preparation: Tincture made by dissolving one part of camphor gum in 9 parts of Alcohol.

It was proved by Hahnemann recording 344 symptoms (MMP Vol. IInd Ed.) (Pierce-340).

II. General Analysis (Cow.)

Acts powerfully upon Cerebro-spinal system causing general prostration, giddiness, convulsion, epileptiform, and other nervous systems. In mucous tissues, gives rise to coryza, and diarrhoea. Though its primary action upon stomach is of extreme coldness and torpor of those parts, the system is found in profound collapse, body being ice cold. The genital organs being cold and relaxed, in urinary tract strangary is established. Its action is rapid and intense. Chief sphere of usefulness-cholera, cold-effects of.

III. Suited to (Allen-79)

Persons physically and mentally weak and irritable. Exceedingly sensitive to cold air (Hep. s., Kali m., Psor.). Pain better while thinking of it (Bell.-worse, Calc. phos., Helon. d., Oxal. ac.).

IV. Clinical (Clarke I-370)

Angina pectoris, Bed-sores, Cholera asiatica, Chordee, Colds, Convulsions, Epilepsy, Eruptions suppressed, Erysipelas, Gonorrhoea, Heart affections, Hyperpyrexia, Influenza, Measles, Memory lost, Priapism, Rheumatism, Sexual mania, Shivering, Sleeplessness, Snake-bites, Spasms, Strangury, Sunstroke, Taste disordered, Tetanus, Tobacco-habit, Twitching, Urethra-spasmodic stricture of, Urine-suppression of.

V. **Symptoms-General** (Nash 398-399)

1. Great coldness of the external surface, with sudden and complete prostration of the vital force; collapse.
2. The patent objects to being covered, not withstanding the objective coldness; throws off all the covering.
3. Pains disappear when thinking of them; exceedingly sensitive to cold air.

VI. **Symptoms-Particular** (Nash-399)

1. Cholera TRIO of Hahnemann of which Camph.. is the chief Remedy.

   Camph.-Collapse with painless or no stools. Great external coldness. wants no cover (Sec.).

   Verat. -Collapse as consequence of profuse evacuation of stomach & bowel, cold sweat on forehead with great external coldness.

   Cupr. -when cramp in stomach and extremities.
2. Collapse-great coldness of body with sudden and complete prostration of vital forces.

VII. **Black Letter Symptoms** (Tyler-176)

- Better when thinking of the existing complaint.
- Throbbing, like beats with a hammer, in cerebellum, 150-chronous with pulse, head hot, face red, limbs cool, in standing; mostly with such as were deprived of sexual intercourse.
- Contraction as if laced together in cerebellum and glabella, with coldness all over. Very sensitive to cold air.
- Nose cold and pointed (in Diarrhoea and Cholera).
- Cold sweat, with vomiting.

- Tongue, cold, flabby, trembling.
- Anxiety and restlessness, absence of evacuations, frequently chilly or feeling as if cold air was blowing on covered parts; great sinking and collapse (cholera).
- Burning during urination.
- Newborn children; asphyxia; hard places in skin on abdomen and thighs, quickly increasing and getting hardened, sometimes with a deep redness spreading nearly over whole abdomen and thighs; violent fever, with startings and titanic spasms, with bending backward; they make no water.
- Influenza.
- Cool breath, as from grave, playing upon hand held before mouth-Carb. v. Coldness of limbs.
- Congestion to Chest. All sequels of measles.
- Cold, clammy, weakening sweat.
- Pulse-weak, imperceptible; frequent and scarcely perceptible; accelerated, without fever; very much accelerated, but undulating and without strength; very rapid; full and rapid; full and irritable; irritable in evening; hard or soft; extremely small and slow; small and hard, becoming slower and slower; small, weak and quite frequent; couldn't be counted; Icy coldness all over, with death-like paleness of face. Diminished circulation to parts most distant from heart. Effects of shocks from injury; surface of body cold; face pale and bluish, lips livid; diarrhoea; pulse feeble, nervous anxiety and stupefaction; signing respiration; great exhaustion.

CANNABIS INDICA

I. Introduction (Cow.-185)

Natural Order: Urticaceae.
Common Name: Indian Hemp, Hashish.
Habitat: A native plant of India, Botanically same as Cannabis sativa, but possessing very different medicinal properties.
Preparation: Tincture from the dried herb topes.

It was proved by Hahnemann recording 330 symptoms in MMP Vol. I. Most extensive provings of this drug were made by the American Provers' Union and published in 1839 (Pierce-334).

II. General Analysis (Cow.)

Acts as a powerful excitant of nervous system, increasing both intellectual and motor activity. For this reason, is used in India as an intoxicating exhilarant. Its action depends largely upon the temperament of the individual.

III. Suited to (Allen-80)

Very forgetful person, forgets his last words, laughs immoderately. Laughs and cries alternately. Inability to recall any thought or event, on account of other thoughts in mind (Anac., Lac can.).

IV. Clinical (Clarke-I-376)

Catalepsy, Chordee, Clairvoyance, Delirium tremens, Delusions, Epilepsy, Gonorrhoea, Headache, Mania, Menorrhagia, Paralysis, Prostatitis, Satyriasis, Stammering, Uraemia, Urinary disorders.

V. Symptoms-General (Nash-458)

1. Patient can't complete his sentence, so forgetful. She is unable to talk.

VI. Black Letter Symptoms (Tyler-182)

- Imagines he hears music; shuts his eyes and is lost for some time in the most delicious thoughts and dreams.
- Incoherent talking.
- Fixed ideas.
- Exaltation of spirits, with excessive loquacity.
- Laughs immoderately.
- Uncontrollable laughter, till face becomes red and the back and Ions ache.
- Anguish accompanied by great oppression, ameliorated in the open air. He was in constant fear he would become insane.
- Very absent-minded.
- Every few moments he would lose himself, and then wake up, as it were, to those around him.
- Vertigo.
- Frequent involuntary shaking of the head.
- On regaining consciousness, violent shocks pass through his brain.
- Fixed gaze.
- Infection of the vessels of the conjunctiva of both eyes.
- While reading, the letters run together.
- Throbbing and fullness in both ears.
- Ringing and buzzing in the ears.
- He looks drowsy and stupid.
- His lips are glued together.
- Dryness of the mouth and lips.
- White, thick, frothy, and sticky saliva.
- The throat is parched, accompanied by intense thirst for cold water.
- Increased appetite.
- Ravenous hunger.
- Pain in the cardiac orifice.
- Burning and scalding before, during and after urination.
- Stinging pain before, during and after urination.
- Profuse colourless urine.
- The urine dribbles out after the stream ceases.

- On squeezing the glans penis, a white glairy mucus oozes out.
- Satyriasis.
- Rough cough, which scratches the breast under the sternum.
- Pulse below the natural standard, as low as 46.
- Pain across the shoulders and spine, forcing him to stoop, and preventing him from walking erect.
- Paralysis of the lower extremities and right arm.
- Agreeable thrilling through the arms and hands.
- Entire paralysis of the lower extremities.
- Agreeable thrilling in both limbs from the knees down, with a sensation as if a bird's claws were clasping the knees.
- Thoroughly exhausted from a short walk.
- Excessive sleepiness.
- Sound sleep.
- Profuse sticky sweat, standing out in drops on his forehead.

CANNABIS SATIVA

I. Introduction (Cow.-189)

Natural Order: Urtricaceae.
Common Name: Hemp.
Habitat: Native of Europe and America, an annual dioecious plant.
Preparation: Tincture from fresh herb tops.

It was first proved by Hahnemann (Pierce-346).

II. General Analysis (Cow.)

Acts esp. Upon mucous lining of the urinary tract, prepuce, giving rise to excessive irritation, followed by inflammation and mucous discharges similar to Gonorrhoea . Mental activity of Cann. sat. is far reduced than Cann. ind. and other effects due to different other constituents of the plant (Eatherial oil, Potash Nitrate).

III. Suited to (Allen-81)

Sensation of drops of water falling on or from single parts; on head, from anus, stomach, heart. Urethral and related complaints with asthma and constipation (even without these), very sensitive to touch. Obstinate constipation, causing retention of urine; constriction of arms.

IV. Clinical (Clarke-I-380)

Ascites, Asthma, Cataract, Cystitis, Eyes-corneal opacity, Fingers contracted, Gonorrhoea, Headache, Hysteria, Infantile leucorrhoea, Nephritis, Nose-bleed, Palpitation, Phimosis, Pleurisy, Pneumonia, Post-partum haemorrhage, Priapism, Stammering, Tetanus, Trachea-mucus in, Urethral caruncle.

V. Symptoms-Particular (Nash-313)

1. Urethra- irritation, inflammation.
2. Urinary tract. Very strong action on the urinary organs.
3. Urethra very sensitive to touch or external pressure. He can't walk with legs together. Severe back pain if the disease has extended up to the urethra or bladder, every few minutes, may be bloody urine.
4. Sense of dropping in or near area of heart.
5. Gonorrhoea -one of the best medicines in.

Merc. c.	—thick green discharge
Puls. or Sep.	—thick and bland discharge.
Sul.	—Gleet.

CANTHERIS

I. Introduction (Cow-191)

Synonym: Cantheris Vasicatoria
Common Name: Spanish fly.
Preparation: Tincture made from dried flies by digesting in alcohol.

Hahnemann first introduced this medicine in Homeopathy, but recorded only 105 symptoms. It was further proved by others and Allen's Encyclopædia records 1651 symptoms. (Pierce-347).

II. General Analysis (Cow.)

Acts chiefly upon mucous membranes and the skin. In the former its most decisive action is upon the mucous lining of the urinary tract, where it produces from an irritation to destructive inflammation of either part or the whole tract. Upon the skin it causes erysipelous form of inflammation. Even sloughing blisters. Chief characteristics-constant urge to urinate, scanty discharge, violent cutting, burning pains before, during and after urination.

III. Suited to (Allen-82)

Over sensitiveness of all parts. Haemorrhage from all outlets, Pain-raw sore, burning in every part of the body, internally and externally. Constant urging to urinate, passing but a few drops at a time mixed with blood (sudden desire to urinate and intense itching in urethra-Petrosel.) Intolerable urging before, during and after urination, violent pains in bladder, burning acting pains in urethra while urinating, violent tenesmus and strangury sexual desire increased in both sexes. Preventing sleep, violent priapism with excessive pain. (Pic. ac.)

IV. Clinical (Clarke I-383)

Bladder affections, Burns, Chordee, Diphtheria, Dysentery, Eczema, Emissions, Erotomania, Erysipelas, Eyes inflamed, Gastritis, Gonorrhoea , Herpes zoster, Hydrophobia, Kidney-affections of, Mania, Neuralgia, Nymphomania, Ovaries-affections of, Peritonitis, Placenta retained, Pleurisy, Pregnancy-affections of, Satyriasis, Scarlatina, Spermatorrhoea, Strangury, Thirst, Throat sore, Tongue-inflammation of, Urine abnormal, Vesication of skin.

V. Symptoms-General (Nash-147)

1. Frequent urge to urinate-straining and cutting, burning pains. Small unsatisfactory quantity passed at a time, or bloody urine.
2. Excessive burning pains. (eyes, mouth, throat, stomach, intestinal tract; all the mucous surfaces and skin).
3. Stringy and tenacious discharge from the mucous membrane.
4. Nearly all complaints accompanied with the characteristic urinary symptoms.
5. Erysipelas, with blebs or large blisters filled with water and burning pain; useful for surface burns. (locally).
6. Uncontrollable anguish, furious rage, frenzied delirium; strong sexual desire, both sexes.
7. Disgust for everything; drink; food tobacco.
8. Dysenteric stools, bloody and shreddy, like scrapings from intestines, with tenesmus in rectum and bladder.

VI. Symptoms-Particular (Nash-147-51)

1. Urinary organs-Centre of action.
2. Strong action upon skin and urinary organs.
3. AIR PASSAGE with tenacious mucous with urinary symptoms

   Canth.,

   Hydras.,

Kali bich.,
Coc. cact. etc.

4. Few symptoms related to urinary organs are—violent pain in bladder with frequent urging to urinate, with intolerable tenesmus, before, during and after urinating—fearful cutting pains in the urethra. Constant urging to urinate, urine passed in drops with extreme pains in the urethra. Urine scalds and is passed in drops.
5. Skin—
   (i) ERYSIPELAS
   Apis.—more oedema and stinging with urinary irritation.
   Canth.—more blister and burning.
   Ars.—Great thirst with intense burning.
   (ii) BURNS AND BURNING
   Canth. } both externally and internally blebs or watery.
   Ars. } vesicles from which burn and itch.

VII. Black Letter Symptoms (Tyler-197)

- Great amativeness; amorous frenzy.
- Inflammation of eyes, particularly when caused by a burn.
- Burning sensation in throat which feels as if on fire.
- Passage of white or pale red though mucous with stool, like scrapings from intestines, with streaks of blood.
- Paroxysmal cutting and burning pains in both Kidneys, the region very sensitive to slightest touch, alternating with pain in tip of penis; urging to urinate; painful evacuation, by drops of bloody urine, and at times, of pure blood.
- Violent tenesmus in vesicae and strangury.
- Painful discharge of a few drops of bloody urine, causing very severe sharp pain, as if a red-hot iron was passing along urethra; this pain was most cutely felt at membranous portion of canal, and in meatus urinaritus.

- Violent burning, cutting pains in neck of bladder, extending to fossa navicularis, < before and after urinating.
- Violent pains in bladder with frequent urging; intolerable tenesmus.
- Urging to urinate from smallest quantity of urine in bladder.
- Dribbling discharge, reddish, sometimes mixed with blood.
- Ardor urinae.
- Before, during, and after urinating fearful cutting pains in urethra; she must double herself and scream pains.
- Burning, when urinating, and when not.
- Retention of urine, causing pain. Suppressed gonorrhoea.
- Sexual desire; increased; disturbing sleep at night.
- Frightful satyriasis; violent, painful priapism, with excessive pains.
- Retained placenta or membranes, usually with painful urination.
- Burning in chest.
- Pain in loins, with incessant desire to urinate.
- Pain in loins, Kidneys and abdomen, with such pain on urinating that he could not pass a single drop without moaning and screaming.
- In third stage, when there is complete insensibility; Cramp in abdomen, muscles and legs; suppression of urine; Haemorrhage from stomach and intestines; cold sweat on hands and feet (Yellow fever).
- Scalds and Burns.
- Burns, before blisters form, and when they have formed.

CAPSICUM

I. Introduction (Cow-196)

Synonym: Capsicum Annum.
Natural Order: Solanaceae.
Common Name: Cayenne, red pepper.
Habitat: A herbaceous plant cultivated almost in every part of the world.
Preparation: Tincture from ripe dried fruit.

It was first proved by Hahnemann recording 340 symptoms (MMP Vol. 1) (Pierce-349).

II. General Analysis (Cow.)

Acts upon mucous membranes and causes intense irritation to congestion and inflammation upon mucous membranes of respiratory tract and alimentary canal. Produces ulcers, abscess, phlegmonous condition like Canth., is eliminated through kidneys causing inflammation and strangury tenesums etc. Chief feature of Caps. is sensation of intense burning and smarting as if it pepper has been sprinkled upon the parts.

III. Suited to (Allen-83)

Persons with light hair, blue eyes, nervous but stout and plethoric habit. Phlegmatic (emotionally stable) diathesis, lack of reactive power, esp. with fat people; easily exhausted, dreads exercise of any kind, Inclined to be jovial, yet get angry at trifles. Children dread open air, always chilly clumsy, fat, dirty. Home sickness with sleeplessness. Desires to be left alone, wants to lie down and sleep.

IV. Clinical (Clarke-I-388)

Amaurosis, Asthma, Brain-irritation of, Cough, Delirium tremens, Diarrhoea, Diphtheria, Dysentery, Ear affections,

Glandular swellings, Haemorrhoids, Headache, Heartburn, Hernia, Homesickness, Intermittents, Lung affections, Measles, Mouth ulcerated, Neuralgia, Nose affections, Obesity, Oesophagus-constriction of, Paralysis, Pleuro-pneumonia, Pregnancy-affections of, Rectum-diseases of, Rheumatic gout, Rheumatism, Sciatica, Scrofula, Sea-sickness, Stomatitis, Throat sore, Tongue-paralysis of, Trachea-tickling in, Urine-disorders of, Whooping-cough, Yellow fever.

V. **Symptoms-General** (Nash-418)

1. Burning pains especially in mucous membranes or smarting as from red pepper on the parts.
2. Cough with pain in distant parts as head, bladder, knees, legs etc.
3. Chill or shuddering after every drink, begins between shoulders and spreads all over.

VI. **Symptoms-Particular** (Nash-418)

1. Burning in mucous membranes in any area.
   Ars.-better hot application.
   Caps.-No relief from heat, as if red pepper applied to affected part.
2. Headache-Cough, holds head, as if it would burst when coughing.
   > lying, sitting <
   Bry.,
   Nat. m.,
   Squil.,
   Sul.
3. Pain, on coughing, in bladder, knee, leg etc.
4. Chill-begins between shoulders and spreads after every drink. Lack of reaction especially in fat people.

VII. **Black Letter Symptoms** (Tyler-200)

- Home sickness.
- Of a contented disposition; is jocular and sings, and yet on slightest cause gets angry.

- Disposition to start. After emotions, fever with red cheeks.
- Intoxication.
- Confusion of head; or, all the senses are more acute.
- When moving head and when walking, headache as if the skull would burst.
- Throbbing, beating headache; in one of the temples; in the forehead. Pressive pain in forehead.
- Drawing, tearing pain, left side of head.
- As if cayenene pepper were sprinkled on parts.
- Burning in skin.
- Haemorrhoidal constitutions.
- A shooting headache, worse at rest, better by movement.
- An outstretching headache, as if the brain were too full.
- Drawing, tearing pains in frontal bone, more on right side.
- Aching pain in eyes as from a foreign body.
- Swellings, of Mastoid process; Painful to touch.
- Periostitis and Caries of mastoid.
- Tearing pain in concha of ear.
- An itching or aching pain quite deep in ear.
- Epistaxis.
- Burning blisters in Mouth.
- Tough mucous in mouth: or dryness.
- Taste foul: like putrid water.
- Chaps on the lips: fissured lips.
- Tough mucous in posterior nares on rising: difficult to dislodge.
- Tonsilitis, with burning, smarting pain.
- Great soreness in throat, with smarting.
- Pain when swallowing, burning and other pains in throat, worse between acts of swallowing.
- Throat inflamed, dark-red, burning, pressing.
- Heartburn.
- Dyspepsia from torpidity; especially in old people.
- Stomach ice cold: or burning in stomach.
- Inclined to vomit.

- Thirst: drinking causes shuddering; drawing pains in back.
- Burning, cutting pains in ABDOMEN.
- After every stool, thirst, and after every drink shivering.
- Aching tension, ABDOMEN, especially in stomach, worse movement: with aching tension lower part of back.
- Tensive pain, abdomen to chest, as from distension.
- Abdomen feels distended almost to bursting, impeding breathing to suffocation.
- A drawing and turning over in abdomen.
- After flatulent colic in hypogastrium, small frequent stools of mucous mixed with blood, which cause tenesmus.
- Tenesmus: violent tenesmus.
- Burning pain in anus.
- Dysentery: tenesmus and stranguary: pain worse from a current of air, even if warm.
- Smarting and burning pain in the anus and rectum.
- Tenesmus of rectum and bladder at the same time.
- Relaxed fibre-obesity.
- Shuns all movements.
- Haemorrhoids, burning as if pepper were sprinkled on them, swollen, itching, throbbing: with sore feeling in anus: bleeding or blind with mucous discharge; with bloody mucous stools; with drawing pain in back and cutting pain in abdomen.
- Small frequent stools of mucous, at times with blood: cause tenesmus.
- Burning in bladder.
- Burning, smarting after urination.
- STRANGURY: tenesmus neck of BLADDER: urging to frequent, almost ineffectual urination.
- Scalding of urine.
- Gonorrhoea: second stage: white discharge: excessive sensibility of parts to contact: chordee only suppressed by cold water.
- Creeping and tickling in NOSE, as in stuffed coryza.

- Hoarseness; from straining voice, in singers, preachers, etc.
- When coughing, headache as if skull would burst.
- COUGH expels an offensive breath from lungs.
- Nervous, spasmodic cough.
- Tightness of CHEST: appears to come out of stomach.
- Chest constricted, with oppressed breathing: worse very slight movement.
- Throbbing pain in chest.
- Drawing tearing pain in and near spine.
- Tensive pain in knee.
- Coldness beginning in back.
- Shivering.
- Lack of reactive force, especially in fat people.
- Is wide awake at night: can't sleep.
- Sleep full of dreams.
- Yawning.
- Great desire to lie down and sleep.
- So awkward that she runs into everything.
- Sea-Sickness.
- Lazy, fat, unclean persons who dread open air.
- Children who are always chilly.
- Shivering with chilliness after every drink.

CARBO ANIMALIS

I. Introduction (Cow-199)

Common Name: Animal Charcoal.
Preparation: Trituration of charred Ox-hide.

It was proved by Hahnemann in 1827(Pierce-352). Among the carbon derived from the all kingdoms, vegetable, animal, mineral, it is the least used one. He recorded its 725 symptoms (Chronic Diseases Vol I).

II. General Analysis (Cow.)

Acts mainly upon glandular system and digestive organs; in the former producing painful swellings, inflammation and ulcers, and in the later, symptoms of dyspeptic (indigestion) nature, Glandular action often of a scirrhous nature is its most marked feature.

III. Suited to (Allen-85)

Elderly persons with marked nervous plethora, blue cheeks, blue lips, and great debility, persons with headache as if a tornado in head; as if head had been blown to pieces. Easily strained from lifting; ankles turn when walking.

IV. Clinical (Clarke-392)

Acne rosacea, Aneurism, Appetite disordered, Breast-cancer of, Bubo, Cancer, Cataract, Constipation, Coccygodynia, Cough, Empyaema, Eructations, Face-eruption on, Gangrene, Glandular indurations, Haemorrhoids, Headache, Homesickness, Hypertrophy, Lactation-effects of, Legs-pain in, Leucorrhoea, Lumbago, Nose affections, Otorrhoea, Pancreas indurated, Perspiration altered, Pleurisy, Polypi, Scrofula, Strabismus, Syphilis, Tongue-affections of, Trachea-affections of, Ulceration, Uterus-cancer of, Vision disordered.

V. **Symptoms-Particular** (Nash-251)

1. Great weakness/prostration in persons who are disposed to glandular swellings, indurations, suppurations.
2. Old suppurating Bubo-Lach., Tarent. cub..
3. Copper colour skin eruption.
4. Weak ankles in children-Carb. a., Nat. c., Sel.
5. Menses too early and too long. Flow always weakens, so that she can hardly speak.
6. Menorrhogia from chronic induration of uterus,. also in catchetic women with glandular swellings.

CARBO VEGETABILIS

I. Introduction (Cow.-203)

Common Name: Vegetable charcoal.
Preparation: Trituration of the charcoal made from birch or beech wood.

It was proved by Hahnemann. It first appeared in MMP, along with Carbo. a. In Chronic Diseases he recorded its 1185 symptoms (Pierce-355).

II. General Analysis (Cow.)

Chief action is upon the mucous membranes of digestive tract (causing excessive accumulation of gas) and the stomach and bowels, upon blood devitalising it; and upon nervous system exhausting it. Chief action-causing excessive accumulation of the gas in bowels and stomach.

III. Suited to (Allen-86)

Bad effects of exhausting diseases (China, Phos. Psor.). Bad effects of previous illness, injury, typhoid (Psor.). Ailments-quinine, Mercury, salt, spoiled fish, fat, getting over heated (Ant. c.). Loss of fluids (Caust.), bleeding (China, Phos.) Loose teeth, Easily bleeding gum, Excessive gas-eructations give temporary relief, persons who have never fully recovered from the exhausting effects of some previous illness; asthma after measles or pertussis of childhood, Indigestion from drunken debauch, etc.

IV. Clinical (Clarke-I-397)

Acidity, Acne, Angina pectoris, Aortitis, Aphonia, Asthenopia, Asthma, Breasts-erysipelas of, Bronchitis, Burns, Carbuncles, Catarrh, Chilblains, Cholera, Constipation, Cough, Deafness, Debility, Diarrhoea, Distension, Dysentery, Dyspepsia, Emphysema, Erysipelas, Eructations, Feet cold,

Flatulence, Gangrene, Haemorrhage, Haemorrhoids, Hair falling off, Headache, Heart disease, Influenza, Intermittents, Intertrigo, Irritation, Laryngitis, Lungs congested, Measles, Mumps, Nose-bleed, Oesophagitis, Orchitis, Otorrhoea, Pregnancy-affections of, Purpura, Scabies, Scurvy, Shivering, Sleep disordered, Starting, Stomach disordered, Stomatitis, Trachea-dryness of, Tympanites, Typhus, Ulcer, Yellow fever.

V. **Symptoms-General** (Nash-52)

1. Vital force nearly exhausted; complete collapse.
2. Blood stagnates in the capillaries; veinous turgescence; surface cold, blue.
3. Haemorrhages (nose, stomach, gums, bowels, bladder or any mucous surface), with indescribable paleness of the surface of the body.
4. Mucous membranes break down, become spongy, bleed, ulcerate and become putrid.
5. Excessive flatulence, pressing upward stomach and abdomen.
6. Hunger for oxygen, decarbonized blood; cries, "fan me, fan me hard".
7. Anaemic, especially after acute diseases, which has greatly depleted the patient ; chronic effects.
8. Person who has never fully recovered from the exhausting effec\\ts of some previous illness; has never recovered from effects of typhoid, weak digestion; the simplest food disagrees, erucations give temporary relief.
9. Bad effects from loss of vital fluids (Caust.); haemorrhage from any broken down condition of mucous membrane.
10. Looseness of teeth, easily bleeding gums.
11. In the last stages of disease, with copious cold sweat, cold breath, cold tongue, voice lost, this remedy may save a life.
12. Coldness of the knees, even in bed (Apis.) of left arms and leg. Very cold hands and feet; fingernails blue.
13. Persons who have never recovered from effects of some previous illness or injury, suppression by Quinine or drugging, typhoid or yellow fever.

14. China is its great complementary.

VI. **Symptoms-Particular** (Nash-53-57)

1. Vital forces nearly exhausted. Cold surface, esp. from knees to feet, motionless, breath cold, pulse intermittent, cold sweat on limbs. Debilitated condition. (Carb. v., Ars., Mur. ac.).
2. Gums spongy, bleed on touching or sucking them or become retracted from teeth, sore or sensitive on chewing or when pressing together.
3. Flatulence in stomach, < lying down (KEY).
4. Whole alimentary canal deeply affected with broken down condition. Stomach weak. Acidity and pyrosis frequent. Plain food, esp. fat disagrees (Puls.). Suceeds when Puls. fails.
5. Depressing influence of some prior derangement.
   Carb. v.,
   Psor.,
   Rhus t., physical strain since.
   Calc. c.
6. Complaint from excessive burning in stomach-upper part of abdomen, of flatulence.
7. Bronchitis of old people.
8. Chest-burning as from glowing coal, weak feeling in
   Carb. v.,
   Phos. ac.,
   Stan.,
   Sul.
9. Haemorrhage-from broken down condition of mucous membranes (lungs, nose, stomach, bowels, bladder etc.).
10. Hoarseness < damp air esp. evening. (morning hoarseness-Caust.).

VII. **Black Letter Symptoms** (Tyler-211)

- Indifference; heard everything without feeling pleasantly or unpleasantly and without thinking of it.
- Anxiety: as if oppressed with heat in face; accompanied by shuddering; on closing eyes; in evening, after lying down; on awakening.

- Fainting after sleep; after rising, or while yet in bed, morning belching; caused by debilitating losses, or abuse of mercury.
- Dull headache in occiput; violent pressive pain in lower portion of occiput feeling of weight.
- Head feels heavy as lead.
- Hat pressed upon head like a heavy weight, and he continued to feel the sensation even after taking it off, as if head was bound up with a cloth.
- Sweat on forehead, often cold.
- Burning in eyes.
- Parotitis.
- Looseness of teeth, with bleeding of gums, which are very sensitive.
- Tongue turns black.
- Tongue cold.
- Stomacace.
- Great accumulation of flatus in stomach.
- Stomach feels tense and full; flatulence.
- Distension of stomach and abdomen.
- Burning in Rectum.
- Itching of anus.
- Rawness and chafing of children in hot weather.
- Cholera asiatica, stage of collapse.
- After sexual excesses and onanism.
- Soreness, itching, and burning and swelling of pudenda.
- Debility from nursing. Gastralgia.
- Great roughness in larynx, with deep, rough voice, which failed if he exerted it, through without pain in throat.
- Breathing short, with cold hands and feet.
- Desires to be fanned, must have more air.
- Weak, fatigued feeling of chest, particularly on waking.
- Pneumonia: third stage, foetid sputum; cold breath and sweat; wants to be fanned; threatened paralysis of lungs.
- Fine itching eruption on Hands.
- Cold knees, particularly in night.

- Ulcer on leg burns at night, discharge offensive, mottled, purple.
- Awakens often from Cold limbs, especially cold knees.
- Adynamic and gastric fever, occurring in hot weather from abuse of ice water and other summer beverages.
- Typhoid and yellow fever patients; cyanotic, and coldness of limbs, almost in agony of death; impending paralysis of heart and collapse.
- Yellow fever, third stage, Haemorrhage, with great paleness of face, violent headache, great heaviness in limbs and trembling of body.
- Swelling of glands, in scrofulous or syphilitic persons.
- Sepsis, sunken features, sallow complexion, hectic, typhoid symptoms.
- Blue colour of body, with terrible cardiac anxiety and icy coldness of whole surface (Cyanosis).
- Ulcerations, with burning pain.
- Vital powers low, Veinous system predominant.

CAULOPHYLLUM

I. Introduction (Cow-213)

Synonym: Caulophyllum Thalictroides.
Natural Order: Berberidaceae.
Habitat: A perennial herb growing in rich woods in most part of the US.
Common Name: Blue Cohosh, Papoose Root.
Preparation: Tincture from fresh root.

It was first proved by Dr. Burt but its thorough and complete proving is still awaited (Pierce-361).

II. General Analysis (Cow.)

Acts upon muscular tissue of female generative organs, and especially upon uterine motor nerves, also upon small muscles and joints.

III. Suited to (Allen-89)

Women-ailments of, during pregnancy, parturition, lactation. Rheumatism of women, esp., of small joints. (Act. rac.), erratic pains changing place every few minutes (Puls.); Painful stiffness of affected joints.

IV. Clinical (Clarke I-430)

Abortion threatened, After-pains, Amenorrhoea, Barrenness, Bearing-down pains, Chloasma, Cholera morbus, Dysmenorrhoea, False conception, Feet-affections of, Gonorrhoea, Hand-affections of, Inframammary pain, Labour-abnormal; false pains of, Leucorrhoea, Menstruation disordered, Ovarian neuralgia, Pityriasis, Pregnancy-affections of, Rheumatic gout, Rheumatism, Uterine spasm, Uterine atony.

V. Symptoms-General (Nash-213)

1. Metrorrhagia-flow of dark and liquid, of passive nature, great sense of internal trembling and weakness.
2. Very valuable women's remedy. Long continued passive haemorrhage after miscarriage.
3. Regulates irregular spasmodic labour pains. Also relieves pains of same character in dysmenorrhoea.

CAUSTICUM

I. Introduction (Cow.-215)

Preparation: A mixture of Caustic Lime and Bisulphate of Potash, probably a weak solution of Potassium Hydrate. First three lowest decimal dilutions made with dilute alcohol, then with alcohol.

The drug was first recorded in MMP editions but Hahnemann transferred its pathogenesis to Chronic Diseases Vol. I recording 1505 symptoms (Chronic Diseases Vol. I) (Pierce-364).

II. General Analysis (Cow.)

It produces paralysis of vocal organs, with inflammation of mucous lining, larynx and trachea. It causes paralysis of all muscles of face, paresis (slight Paralysis) of sphincter vasicae, and other single parts. Paralytic weakness and general weakness of all potash salts. Aphonia (loss of voice) in Laryngeo-tracheal catarrh and paralytic affections are chief spheres of action.

III. Suited to (Allen-91)

Persons with dark hair and rigid fibre, weakly, psoric, with excessively yellow, sallow complexion; subject to affections of respiratory and urinary tracts. Children with dark hair and eyes, delicate, sensitive skin, prone to intertrigo during dentition (Lyc.); or convulsion with eruption of teeth (Stan.).

IV. Clinical (Clarke-I-432)

Acne rosacea, Agalactia, Amaurosis, Apoplexy, Arthritis deformans, Bladder affections, Bronchitis, Burns, Cataract, Chorea, Coccygodynia, Constipation, Convulsions, Cough, Deafness, Dentition, Diphtheritic paralysis, Ear-otorrhoea, Emaciation, Enuresis, Epilepsy, Eyes-affections of, Facial paralysis, Fistula, Fistula dentalis, Goitre, Haemorrhoids, Headache, Heart affections, Heel blistered, Herpes zoster, Hip disease, Hydrogenoid constitution, Impotence, Influenza, Intermittent fever, Intertrigo, Laryngitis, Lead poisoning, Leucorrhoea, Locomotor ataxy, Meniere's disease, Menstruation disordered, Myalgia, Nails crippled, Neuralgia, Nose-crusts in; acne on, Paralysis, Pemphigus, Pregnancy, Prostatitis, Ptosis, Rheumatism, Scabies, Scrofula, Skin-eruptions on, Small-pox, Stammering, Syphilis, Tendons contracted, Throat-affections of, Tongue-affections of; paralysis of, Ulcer, Urethritis, Urinary disorders, Veins-varicose, Voice lost, Warts, Whooping-cough.

V. **Symptoms-General** (Nash-268)

1. Great weakness, faintlike goneness, culminating in local paralysis (vocal organs, tongue, muscles of deglutition, eyelids, face, bladder and extremities).
2. Obstinate neuralgias, especially of psoric origin; pains of a cramping, drawing nature.
3. Sensation of sore rawness (scalp, throat, larynx and trachea, chest, rectum, anus, urethra and Eruption with burning).
4. Contractions of the ligaments (arthritis deformans).
5. Dry cough with pain in hip and involuntary urination.
6. Soreness and rawness in air passages, can't raise the mucous, < on expiration, > swallowing cold water.
7. Haemorrhoids sore and raw < on walking. Constipation frequent, ineffectual desire for stool; passes better on standing.
8. Modalities: < dry weather, walking (piles), > wet weather, swallowing cold water (cough).

VI. **Symptoms-Particular** (Nash-268-76)

1. Great weakness, faint like, anti Psoric or sinking of strength with trembling.
2. Drooping of eyelids (Sep., Gels., Caust.)

3. Weakness progresses to paralysis.
   Left sided—ach. Right sided—Caust.
   Local paralysis–of vocal organs, muscles of deglutition, of tongue, eyelids, face, bladder etc.
   Nervous twitching, chorea, epileptic attacks, locomotor ataxia.
4. Depression, Sorrow, Melancholy.
   From long lasting grief or sorrow. (Ign., Nat. m., Phos. ac., Caust.)
5. (a) Vision—appearance of a gauze before eyes, or as if a fog after, in case of incipient cataract.
   (b) Ears—Roaring, tickling, all sorts of noises. Best medicine of deafness with noises.
   (c) Voice—Reverberation of sound, esp. of his own. Sul. and Caust. follow each other well.
   (d) Face—Sickly yellow, paralysis prosopoplagia of same origin, stiffness of the Jaw.
6. (a) Throat Burning pain<Swallowing Pain on both sides, Rawness, tickle with dry cough.
   Sul.—burning more on right side.
   (b) Tongue—Paralysis, indistinct speech (Gels.), tongue white coated on sides, middle red.
7. Constipation with little stool.
   Nux. v., Caust.—(Red face with)
   Stool passes better standing-Caust.,
   Haemorrhoids—swollen, itching, wet, worse—walking.
8. Urine—sense of soreness, rawness in urethra, itching of orifice of Urethra, constant ineffectual desire to pass urine (Nux. v., Caust., Canth.) but only a few drops, with spasm in rectum and constipation.
9. Retention of urine. Only few drop occasionally with frequent and urgent desire. Involuntary urine when coughing, sneezing, etc. with deposits at night when asleep; when walking (Bry.). Urinates without sensation of stream, urine loaded with deposits (lithic acid and lithades), thick deposits or sediments of various colours.

10. Chronic Hoarseness worse morning (with loss of voice and rawness). Caust.—Can't speak a loud, hoarseness with deep voice (Drosera).
11. Cough. Sense of Burning, soreness, rawness, can't raise mucus. Cough with pain in hip and involuntary urination.

    Iod., Spon.—sensation of burning

    Caust.—< expiration (Acon.), > swallow of cold water.

    Eup. perf., Rhus t.—In influenza with cough.
12. Backaches, arms, leg; stiffness (Paralysis) (Rheumatic), specific paralysis of both or either lower and upper extremities.

    Caust.–worse rising from a chair
Rhus t.
Sul.
} Chronic Rheumatism Paralysis
13. Sensations (Tearing pains often paroxysmal as in neuralgia of face) Sorenes, Rawness, anywhere and Eruption.

    Arn.—as if bruised.

    Rhus t.—aching soreness in muscles, as if strained in the tendons etc.

    Caust.—Soreness of mucous surfaces as if parts were raw. Burning found everywhere.

    Sul.—itching
Apis.—Stinging
Caust.—Rawness
} Generally Caust. is<in clear fine weather. >damp weather. Nux. v., asthma<dry weather>wet weather.

VII. Black Letter Symptoms
(Tyler-226-30)

- Mental, Hysterical weeping after spasms.
- The least thing makes the child cry.
- Melancholy mood; sadness, hopelessness, from care, grief or sorrow.
- Peevish, irritable, censorious.
- Mental and other ailments from long-lasting grief and sorrow.

- Excessive anxiety. Full of apprehension in the evening.
- Very much vexed.
- Indisposed to work.
- Weakness of memory. Absence of mind.
- Inattentive and absent.
- Rheumatic pains in Head so severe as to cause nausea.
- Tinea capitis in occipital region.
- Inclination to close Eyes; they close involuntarily.
- Sensation of heaviness in upper lid, as if he could not raise it easily. Or as if agglutinated to lower lid and could not be easily loosened.
- Paralysis of eye muscles, especially if from exposure to cold.
- Burning in eyes: visible jerking of the lids.
- Sight obscured, as if a thick fog were before the eyes.
- Incipient Cataract.
- Pressure in eyes as if sand in them.
- Dryness: photophobia.
- Words and steps re-echo in Ears.
- Deafness.
- Accumulation of ear wax, sometimes offensive.
- Dry coryza with stoppage of nose.
- Fluent coryza with pain in chest and limbs.
- Itching tip of nose and alae, as well as inside.
- Pimples, ulcers, crusts on tip of nose; inflamed, swollen, scurfy.
- Old warts on nose.
- Violent bleeding of the nose.
- Acne rosacea on cheeks and forehead, in dispersed groups.
- Paralysis of one side of Face.
- Prosopoplagia and rheumatism of face.
- Warts on face, Yellowness of face.
- Tightness and pain in jaws: difficult to open mouth and to eat.
- Arthritic pains in lower jaw.
- Pain lower back tooth extending to nose and eye.
- Painful looseness and elongation of Teeth.
- Stitching and tearing toothache. Throbbing toothache.

- Pain in sound teeth on drawing on cold air.
- Swelling of gums, readily bleeding and tedious suppuration.
- Frequently recurring abscesses of gums.
- Sore place in the upper part of the palate.
- Stuttering, difficult, indistinct speech.
- Speechlessness from paralysis of organs of speech.
- Tongue coated white on both sides, red in middle.
- Burning pain in Throat, not from swallowing; on both sides, seemed to rise from chest.
- Rawness and tickling in throat with dry cough and some expectoration after long coughing.
- Pain in throat, worse by stooping.
- Must swallow continually, throat feels too narrow.
- Mucus collects in throat, can't be raised hawking; is obliged to swallow it.
- Hawking of mucous, with pain in pit of throat.
- Dryness of throat, constantly obliged to swallow.
- Bread causes pressure in Stomach.
- Violent thirst for many days.
- A swallow of cold water relieves spasms (whooping-cough).
- Sour vomiting followed by sour Eructation.
- Cramp in stomach.
- Pinching, clawing in stomach on deep breathing.
- Haemorrhoids sore, painful, unendurable on walking.
- Haemorrhoids; impeding stool: sticking, burning, painful if touched: when thinking of them: from preaching or straining voice.
- The Stool passes better standing.
- Frequent ineffectual efforts to stool with anxiety and redness of face.
- Pain and strong pulsations in perineum.
- Frequent emission of a large quantity of Urine.
- He urinates so easily that he is not sensible of the stream. Can scarcely believe in the dark that he is urinating till he makes sure with his hand.
- Involuntary passage of urine when coughing, sneezing or blowing the nose at night when asleep.

- Retention with frequent and urgent desire, occasionally a few drops or a small quantity may dribble away.
- Itching orifice of urethra.
- Pressive pain in testicles.
- Nipple sore, cracked, surrounded with herpes.
- Sudden loss of Voice.
- Hoarseness, especially evening, with scraping in the throat.
- Muscles of larynx refuse to perform their function; unable to speak a word in spite of every exertion.
- Cough with sore sensation in a streak down along trachea, where it pains on every paroxysm of cough.
- Shortness of breath.
- Cough with sensation as if he could not cough deep enough to start mucous with tickling and rawness.
- Hollow, racking cough.
- Cough relieved by a swallow of cold water.
- Cough better from bending forward.
- Continual annoying cough, with each cough escape of urine.
- Influenza with tired sensation, limbs as if beaten; rheumatic pain.
- Chest tight; must frequently take a deep breath.
- Soreness in chest.
- Stitches in sternum from deep breathing or lifting.
- Painful compression of chest from both sides towards sternum.
- Sensation (chest) as if clothing were too tight.
- Pulse excited towards evening with orgasm of blood.
- Stiffness and pain in neck and throat, pain in occiput; muscles felt as if bound, could scarcely move head.
- Painful stiffness of Back and sacrum, especially rising from a chair.
- Pressing cramp-like pain in small of back, region of kidneys.
- Bruised or darting pain in coccyx; or dull drawing pain.
- Dull drawing and tearing pain in Arms and Hands.

- Paralysis of right arm with glossoplegia.
- Paralysis of upper extremities.
- Paralysis feeling in right hand.
- Trembling of hands.
- Sensation of fullness in hand, when grasping anything.
- Drawing pains in finger joints.
- Contraction and induration of tendons of fingers.
- Warts on tips of fingers; fleshy warts close to nails.
- Soreness between Thighs, high up.
- Drawing and tearing in thighs, legs, knees and feet: worse open air better in warmth of bed.
- Bruised pain in thighs and legs, mornings in bed.
- Marbled skin of thighs and legs.
- Cracking in knees, when walking or descending.
- Tendons of knees seem too short.
- Gonegra. (Gout of knee joints).
- Gouty tearing in region of Lower Leg, especially in small joints of foot, with swelling.
- Cramp in feet, toes and soles.
- Emaciation of feet.
- Children are slow in learning to walk, with unsteady tottering gait.
- Unsteady walking and easy falling of little children.
- Paralytic weakness of Limbs. Weakness and trembling of limbs.
- Intolerable uneasiness of limbs in evening.
- Nerves. Chorea, even at night, right side of face and tongue may be paralysed.
- Weakness and trembling. Faintlike sinking of strength.
- Paralysis: of vocal cords; one sided; of tongue; of eyelids; of face; of extremities; of bladder.
- Gradually appearing paralysis.
- Tearing Pains.
- Terrible sensation of tearing, paroxysmal; often moving forward then remitting, again starting from same spot: neuralgia moving from occiput, upwards and forwards, over vertex.
- Contraction of flexor tendons; tension and shortening of muscle.

- Disturbing functional activity of brain and spinal nerves, resulting in paralysis.
- During first Sleep wets the bed.
- Intense sleepiness, can scarcely resist it, must lie down.
- Yawning and stretching.
- Sleeplessness at night; on account of dry heat. Can't rest in any position.
- Bad effects from night-watching (Cocc.).
- At night he can get no quite position: can't lie still a moment.
- Skin. Sub acute and chronic eruption, similar to blisters from burns.
- Burns and scalds.
- Large, jagged, often pedunculated warts, exuding moisture and bleeding easily.
- Warts and scrofulous affections.
- Varicose and fistulous ulcers.
- Dark-haired persons with rigid fibre most affected.
- Children with black hair and eyes.
- Antidotes poisoning by lead (paralysis). Paralysis of tongue from type held between lips (compositors).
- Abuse of Mercury, and Sulphur in scabies.
- But should remember Causticum in those difficult "Rheumatoid" cases of arthritis where there are deformities and contractions, and the patient suffers more in cold, dry winds, and less on warm, wet days.

CHAMOMILLA

I. Introduction (Cow.-221)

Synonym: Matricaria Chamomilla.
Natural Order: Compositae.
Common Name: Chamomile.
Habitat: An annual plant, (esp. in sandy regions) of Europe.
Preparation: Tincture from fresh flowering plant.

It was proved by Hahnemann who recommended its use in 12th Potency. MMP Vol. I records 493 symptoms (Pierce-371).

II. General Analysis (Cow.)

Primarily acts upon nervous system and motor system. In the former causes intensely acute susceptibility to morbid impressions; in the later causes general exhaustion. Acts prominently upon liver, digestive and respiratory mucous membranes giving rise to congestion, catarrh etc. The leading feature of Cham. is its excessive sensitiveness of pain, accompanied by peevishness and irritability.

III. Suited to (Allen-93)

Persons, especially children, with light brown hair, nervous, excitable temperament, over sensitive due to use or abuse of coffee or narcotics. Children new born, and during period of dentition, peevish, over sensitive to pain, snappish. can't answer civil, quiet only when carried (can't be touched-Ant. c.). Moaning, whining because he can't have what he wants. Driven to despair (Coff.), over sensitive to pain.

IV. **Clinical** (Clarke-I-453)

Acidity, Anger, Asthma (from anger), Blepharospasm, Catarrh, Coffee-effects of, Colic, Convulsions, Cough, Cramps, Croup, Dentition, Diarrhoea, Dysmenorrhoea, Dyspepsia, Earache, Eyes-blepharites; ophthalmia, Eructations, Erysipelas, Excitement, Excoriations, Fainting fits, Fever, Flatulence, Flatulent colic, Gout, Gum-rash, Headache, Hernia, Hysterical joint, Influenza, Jaundice, Lienteria, Labour-disorders of; pains after, Mastitis, Menstruation disordered, Miliary eruption, Milk fever, Miscarriage, Mumps, Neuralgia, Parotitis, Perichondritis, Peritonitis, Pregnancy-affections of, Red-gum, Rheumatism, Salivation (nocturnal), Sciatica, Screaming, Sensitiveness, Spasms, Speech-affections of, Toothache, Ulcer, Uterus-diseases of, Waking-screaming on, Whooping-cough.

V. **Symptoms-General** (Nash-156)

1. Very Irritable Mood; snaps and snarls, will not speak or answer civilly, mad.
2. Exceedingly sensitive to pain, which makes her mad; numbness alternates with, or attends, the pains; sweats with the pains.
3. Excessive uneasiness; anxiety; agonised, tossing about; will only be quieted by carrying the child about.
4. High fever with sweating, especially on the head; thirsty; one check red and hot, the other pale and cold.
5. Dentition diarrhoea ; green stools, foul odour like rotten eggs much colicky pain, abdomen bloated.
6. Cough < dry at night, when asleep from tickling in throat pit; < cold weather and every winter.
7. Especially adopted to children and nervous, hysterical women.
8. Violent rheumatic pains drive him out of bed at night; compel him to walk about.
9. Burning of soles at night; puts feet out of bed Numbness with the pains.

VI. Symptoms-Particular (Nash-156-61)

1. MIND-She knows that she is uncivil, spiteful to her best friends, confesses her fault, then repeats it, says that she can't help it.
2. Nervous Trio-
   Cham.,
   Ign.,
   Coff.
3. Leading anger medicine (Numbness).
   Acon., Bry., Ign., Lyc., Nux. v., Staph., Coloc. One Red
   Other Cold } Cheek.
4. Pain-Leading Remedy with numbness.
   Cham.—excessive sensitive to pain. 'can't bear it', esp. of coffee drinkers. Pain not < heat but not > cold either. Pals > Cold
   Cold air brings troubles.
5. Restlessness.
   Acon., Ars., Rhus t., Cham.
6. Violent Rheumatic pains drive him out and compel him to walk about.
   Cham.—no particular fear, maddened with pain, had rather die.
   Sleeplessness due to pain.
   Rhus t.,
   Ferr.,
   Verat.,
   Bry.—child not to be carried } for keeping him quiet.
   Cham.—to be carried.
7. Few other symptoms in conjunction with peculiar mind and nervous system of this medicine are:
   (i) "Warm sweat on the head wetting the hair".
   (ii) "Pressing earache in spells; tearing pain extorting cries".
   (iii) "Ears particularly sensitive to cold air".
   (iv) "One cheek red and hot, the other pale and cold."
   (v) "Face sweats after eating or drinking".
   (vi) Toothache if anything warm is taken into the mouth (Puls.).

(vii) Toothache recommences when entering a warm room.
(viii) Teeth feel too long.
(ix) Dentition with diarrhoea of green stools smelling like rotten eggs.
(x) Hot and thirsty with the pains; also fainting. (Hep. s.)
(xi) Gastralgia in coffee drinkers; constrictive pain, or as if a stone were in the stomach. (Nux. v.)
(xii) Wind colic; abdomen distended like a drum; wind passes in small quantities without relief.
(xiii) Stools hot, smelling like rotten eggs, corroding (Sul.).
(xiv) Metrorrhagia. Dark, coagulated blood, flowing in paroxysms.
(xv) Menstrual colic, also following anger.
(xvi) Labour pains press upward, or begin in back, and pass off down inner side of thighs.
(xvii) Rigidity of os, pains unendurable.
(xviii) After-pains also unendurable.
(xix) Children have spasms, from fit of anger in the nurse.
(xx) Cough from tickling in throat pit.
(xxi) Cough dry, worse at night, especially while asleep, does not waken when coughing. (Calc. c., Psor.)
(xxii) Chronic cough, worse in winter or cold weather.
(xxiii) Body chilly and cold; face and breath hot.
(xxiv) Heat and chill intermingled (Ars.).
(xxv) Skin moist and burning hot (Bell.).

VII. Black Letter Symptoms

(Tyler-238-42)

- Dullness of senses, diminished power of comprehension.
- Joyless obtuseness of the senses: understands nothing properly, just as if he were prevented doing so by a sort of dullness of hearing, or a waking dream.

- Child cries; quiet only when carried.
- Child does not wish to be touched.
- Very irritable and fretful; child must be carried.
- Piteous moaning of child because he cannot have what he wants.
- Whining restlessness; the child wants this and that, which when offered, is refused or pushed away.
- Averse to talking, short and snappish.
- Cannot endure being spoken to, or interrupted while speaking, especially after rising from sleep.
- Patient cannot bear anyone near him, and answers snappishly.
- Peevish disposition, nothing pleases.
- Peevishness; she seeks a cause for being peevish at everything, can't return a civil answer.
- Irritable, impatient mood.
- Howling on account of a slight, even imaginary insult, which occurred long ago (Staph.).
- Easily chagrined or excited to anger.
- Extreme restlessness, anxious, agonised, tossing about, with tearing pains in abdomen.
- The pains sometimes made him very peevish.
- Over-sensitiveness to pain, which seems unbearable and drives to despair.
- Throbbing Headache, Semi-lateral, drawing, head-ache.
- Transient attacks of throbbing in one half of brain.
- Congestion to head: following anger, with pressure while lying down; on vertex; with heat in face and oppression of chest; with stitches in head and chest.
- (Pain head) increased as soon as attention was directed to it.
- Warm sweat on head, wetting hair.
- Eyes swollen in morning; agglutinated with purulent mucus.
- Violent pressure in orbital region, sensation in eyeball as if it was tightly compressed from all sides, with momentary obstruction of vision.
- Roaring in Ears, as from rushing water.
- Single large stitches in ear, especially when stooping, with ill humour and peevishness about trifles.

- Pressing earache in spells, with tearing pain, extorting cries.
- Particularly sensitive to open air about ears.
- Heat in Face after eating (and sweat).
- Redness of the one Cheek, returning in paroxysms, without shivering or external heat. Hemicrania.
- Red face, or redness and heat of one cheek, the other being pale.
- One cheek red and hot, the other pale and cold.
- Lower lip parts in the middle in a crack (Nat. m., Sep., Graph.)
- Face sweats after eating or drinking.
- On and under tongue, vesicles with shooting pains.
- Toothache if anything warms is taken into Mouth; after coffee, < by talking; in open air, in room; getting warm in bed; during menstruation and pregnancy; most l. side and lower teeth; < at night.
- Toothache recommences when entering the warm room, or drinking anything warm.
- Toothache seems intolerable and makes him very peevish.
- Teeth feel too long.
- Gums red and tender, Dentition.
- Teething children; with watery, greenish, and also chopped diarrhoea, smelling like rotten eggs; jerking of limbs, or starting Convulsion, child bends double and draws legs upon abdomen; moaning; wanting to be carried: dry cough, restless at night; wants to drink; quick rattling breathing.
- Bitter taste in mouth, in morning.
- Heat in mouth, pharynx and oesophagus, to stomach.
- Collection of saliva of metallic, sweetish taste.
- Foetid smell from mouth.
- Spasmodic constriction of pharynx.
- Sore Throat, with swelling of parotid or sub maxillary glands, or tonsil.
- Want of Appetite.
- Great thirst for cold water and desire for acid drinks.

- Likes to hold cold water in mouth for a long time when drinking; dentition.
- After eating and drinking, heat and sweat of face.
- Thirsty and hot with the pains.
- Fruitless efforts to vomit.
- The pains present are aggravated by eructation.
- Pressure in Stomach, as from a stone pressing down.
- Constrictive gastralgia in coffee drinkers.
- Colic returns from time to time, flatus accumulates in hypochondria and stitches shoot through chest. Gurgling in side extending into Abdomen.
- After a meal abdomen becomes distended.
- Wind colic, abdomen distended like a drum, wind passes in small quantities without relief: > by applying warm cloths.
- Children have spasms in consequence of nursing milk vitiated by a fit of anger.
- Abdomen tympanitic and sensitive to touch.
- A white slimy Diarrhoea with bellyache.
- Green watery, corroding, with colic, thirst bitter taste, and bitter Eructation; like chopped or stirred eggs, smelling sour, hot, smelling like rotten eggs; changeable, containing undigested food; mucous and bloody.
- A forcing towards inguinal ring, as if that part too weak, and a hernia would come or constipation from inactivity of rectum.
- Ulcerating Fissure at anus.
- Menstrual colic, following anger.
- Membranous dysmenorrhea.
- Profuse discharge of clotted blood, with sever labour-like pains.
- Drawing from sacral region forward, griping and pinching in uterus, followed by discharge of large clots of blood.
- Yellow, smarting leucorrhoea.
- Labour pains press upward; she is not and thirsty, cross and inclined to scold.
- Rigidity of os; scarcely able to endure the pains.
- After pain, very acute and distressing.

- Pueperal Convulsion, after anger; or has one red cheek, the other being pale.
- Rash of lying in women and nursing infants, caused by heat or errors in diet, with watery, greenish, chopped egg diarrhoea, corroding anus.
- Mammae hard and tender to touch, with drawing pains, is fretful, sleepless and cross.
- Suffocative tightness Chest, Larynx constricted with constant irritation to cough.
- Almost uninterrupted tickling irritation to cough under upper part sternum: does not always result in coughing.
- Tickling in pit of Throat, causing dry, scraping cough, voice hoarse.
- Sensation of rawness and scraping in larynx.
- Hoarseness from viscid mucous in larynx only brought away by violent hawking.
- Suffocative attacks from repercussion of measles eruption, by taking cold.
- Needle-like pricks in Chest: or single severe stitches.
- Asthma after a fit of anger.
- Scraping, dry cough, caused by tickling in pit of throat, < at night, even in sleep, especially with children after taking cold in winter.
- Drawing pain in Back: pain sacrum especially at nights.
- Arms immediately go to sleep, if she grasps anything firmly; she is obliged to let them sink down.
- Cracking in joints, especially lower limbs: pains as if bruised.
- Cramp in legs and calves.
- Burning of soles, at night: puts feet out bed.
- Violent rheumatic pains drive him out of bed at night, and compel him to walk about.
- Sleepless and restless at night.
- Child gets relief from being carried.
- Over-sensitiveness after abuse of coffee or opium.
- Child suddenly stiffens body and bends backwards, kicks when carried screams immoderately and throws everything off. Dentition.

- Tremulous starting up; twitches of limbs and eyelids.
- Single twitches of limbs and of head during morning nap.
- Moaning in sleep, Weeping and howling in sleep. Starts up, cries out, tosses and talks in sleep.
- Sleepy, but can't sleep.
- Pains are aggravated by heat, which relieves abdominal colic.
- Chill and coldness of whole body, with burning heat of face and hot breath.
- Feeling of external heat, without actual external heat.
- Internal heat with shivering.
- Heat and shivering intermingled, mostly with one red and one pale cheek.
- In evening, burning cheeks with transient rigor.
- Burning heat face which comes out of the eyes like fire.
- Long-lasting Heat, with violent thirst; frequent startings in sleep.
- Hot and thirsty with the pains.
- Fever.
- Profuse Sweat of covered parts. (Thuj. of uncovered parts).
- Sweat during sleep, most on head, usually sour smelling.
- Sweat, with smarting sensation in skin.
- Over-sensitiveness of senses, especially if produced by coffee or narcotics.
- Paralytic sensations are always accompanied by drawing or tearing pain, and drawing or tearing pains rarely occur without paralytic or numb sensation in the part.
- Especially helps children new-born and during period of dentition.
- Adults, even aged persons with arthritic or rheumatic diathesis.

CHELIDONIUM MAJUS

I. Introduction (Cow.-226)

Synonym: Chelidonium Majus.
Natural Order: Papaveraceae.
Common Name: Celandine.
Habitat: perennial plant growing in waste places in France and Germany.
Preparation: Tincture from the fresh plant.

Hahneman first proved this medicine for Homeopathy MMP 1 (Pierce-374).

II. General Analysis (Cow.)

Acts powerfully upon hepatic system causing congestion, inflammation, Jaundice, and a train of symptoms indicative of hepatic disturbances. Also acts upon lung (esp. right side) causing congestion, inflammation etc., and symptoms of hepatization. Chief action-constant pain under the lower angle of the right shoulder blade.

III. Suited to (Allen-95)

Persons of light complexion, thin spare irritable. hepatic, gastric, and abdominal complaints. Tongue thickly yellow coated with red edges showing imprint of teeth (Podo.), constant pain under lower and inner angle of right scapula (Kali c., Cheno., Sang., Merc. c.-under the left).

IV. Clinical (Clarke-I-162)

Antrum of Highmore-inflammation of, Cancer, Chest-affections of, Chorea, Constipation, Cough, Diarrhoea, Dyspepsia, Fistula lachrymalis, Gall-stones, Gonorrhoea, Haemoptysis, Haemorrhoids, Headache, Influenza, Jaundice, Laryngismus, Liver-affections of, Nephritis, Neuralgia,

Nose-bleed, Pleurodynia, Pneumonia, Rheumatism, Scald-head, Stiff-neck, Taste disordered, Tumours, Warts, Whooping-cough, Yawning.

V. **Symptoms-General** (Nash-306)

1. Fixed pain (dull or sharp) under lower inner angle of right shoulder blade.
2. Yellow eyes, face, skin, hands, stool clay coloured or yellow, as gold; urine yellow, Tongue thickly coated yellow, with red edges.
3. Right sided remedy; supra-orbital; hypochondriac; lungs; hip; foot cold as ice, etc.

VI. **Symptoms-Particular** (Nash-307-8)

1. Liver, Jaundice, right sided (Lyc.).
2. Fixed pain under inner angle of right shoulder blade is characteristic symptom.
3. Tongue—Thickly coated yellow with red margins, showing imprint of teeth.
4. Liver—pressive pain, obstinate case of Jaundice (Nash-309)—stools grey, clay coloured or gold, yellow as gold. Loss of appetite, nausea or vomiting of bilious matter. Eyes, face, hands skin yellow. Tongue thickly coated yellow-then it is the medicine.
5. Retains nothing but hot drinks in the stomach.
6. Liver Trouble-from simple congestion to inflammation.

VII. **Black Letter Symptoms** (Tyler-249-51)

- Great Laziness and drowsiness, without yawning. Lethargy.
- Great discomfort; feels not at all well, without knowing what is actually the matter with him. Liability and lassitude.
- Distaste for mental exertion and conversation.
- Weary, indolent disposition.
- Vertigo; with bilious vomiting and pain in liver, with stumbling as if to fall forward; on closing eyes, etc.

- Pain over left eye; seemed to press down upper lid.
- Pressive pain right side forehead.
- Heaviness in the occiput.
- Heaviness, sick headaches Neuralgia.
- Curious symptom-cranium feels too small, a forcing in the cerebrum as if it had no room in the skull, and would force through the ear, with noises.
- Right Supra-orbital neuralgia.
- A long-lasting stitch in right Ear.
- Intolerable sensation in both ears, as if wind rushed out of them.
- In both ears, thundering of distant cannon.
- Whites of Eyes dirty yellow.
- Stitches above left eye.
- Increased secretion of meibomian glands.
- Remarkably yellow colour of the Face, especially forehead, nose and cheeks.
- The usual redness of the cheeks has mixture of yellow of a dark colour.
- Greyish yellow sunken countenance.
- Tongue thickly coated yellow with red margin; showing imprint of teeth.
- Mucus in mouth with tough mucous saliva.
- Bitter taste in the mouth.
- Great tension on and in the Throat, above the larynx, as if it were constricted, whereby, however, only the gullet was narrowed.
- Sensation as if the larynx were pressed upon the oesophagus from without, whereby not the breathing but the swallowing was rendered difficult.
- A choking in throat, as if too large a morsel had been too hastily swallowed.
- Loss of Appetite with disgust and nausea.
- Hiccup.
- All complaints lessen after dinner.
- Nausea in hepatitis, and in the vomiting of pregnancy.
- Bilious vomiting.
- Constriction, tension and sensitiveness in pit of Stomach and right hypochondrium.

- A sharp painful stitch in the pit of the stomach which extends through the body to the back.
- Queer sensation, as of an animal wriggling in epigastrium.
- Stitches in region of Liver. Pressive pain, liver.
- Pains from region of liver shooting towards back and shoulder.
- Pains transversely across umbilicus, as if abdomen were constricted by a string.
- Abdominal plethora. Haemorrhoids. Liver affections.
- Continued cutting in Bowels, immediately after eating: food however was relished.
- Diarrhoea and constipation alternately.
- Thin, pasty, bright yellow Stools.
- Urine dark yellow, clear.
- Urine turbid on passing it, brownish-red, like brown beer.
- Urine stains the diaper dark yellow.
- Short, quick Breathing with oppression,>deep inspirations.
- Nightly attacks of asthma with constriction in chest region of diaphragm.
- Hindrance to breathing as by a tight girdle.
- Stitches beneath the right ribs.
- Deep-Seated pain in whole of right side: of Chest.
- Oppression of chest, clothing seemed too tight.
- Soreness in right lower ribs.
- Hepatization of lungs: hoemoptysis; pneumonia.
- Stiffness of Neck.
- Stitches beneath right scapula. Pains in right scapula.
- Stitches: pain, beneath right shoulder blade.
- Tearing lowest lumber Vertebrae, extending to neighbourhood of os ilii; as if vertebrae were broken away from one another, only when bending forwards, and on again bending backwards.
- Pain in right shoulder.
- Tips of fingers cold, yellow, "dead" nails blue; esp. right.
- Drawing pain hips, thighs, legs, feet, especially right side.

- Loss of power left thigh and knee when treading.
- Hard pressure, below both patellae.
- Pain right knee with burning and stiffness < moving.
- Neuralgia in limbs: rheumatism, least touch exceedingly painful; sweat without relief.
- Limbs heavy, stiff and lame: flabby. Tremble and twitch.
- Burning heat of hands, spreads over body.
- Sweat during sleep, after midnight towards morning >waking.
- Tissues. Chronic, gastric and intestinal catarrhs.
- Hepatitis; jaundice; fatty liver, painful enlargement of liver, gall stones; bilious conditions.
- Distension of veins; abdominal plethora; haemorrhoids.
- Yellow grey colour of skin.
- Itching of skin. Red painful pimples and pustules.
- Old, putrid spreading ulcers.

CHENOPODIUM

I. Introduction (Clarke- 1-468)

Common Name: Worn Seed
Natural Order: Chenopodiaceae
Preperation: Tincture of the fresh plant. Solution of Oil Seed.

II. Clinical (Clarke-I-468)

Aphasia, Apoplexy, Asthma, Cerebral deafness, Convulsions, Dropsy, Epilepsy, Headache, Hemicrania, Hemiplegia, Leucorrhoea, Menses suppressed, Paralysis, Scapula-pain in, Tinnitus, Tonsillitis.

III. Symptoms-Particular (Nash-432)

1. Pain under left shoulder-Cheno.
2. Pain under right shoulder-Chel.

} Pain depends upon some hepatic derangements. Chenopodium, Anthrac. and Chelidonium are important for infra-scapular pains.

3. Breast pain (Single symptoms)

Act. rac.— Intra-mammary pains at climacteric.

Crot. t. } Pain from nipple to back when child nurses.
Sil. } Pain in upper left chest though scapula (shoulder blade) (Myrtus com, Pix liquida, Ther., Sul.).

Ars.
Calc. c. } Pain through upper right chest.

Chel.,
Merc. v.,
Kali c. } Pain through lower right chest.

Nat. s. —Pain though lower left chest.

CHIMAPHILLA

I. Introduction (Cow.-230)

Synonym: Chimaphilla Umbelatte.
Natural Order: Ericaceae.
Common Name: Pipsissewe. Prince's Pine.
Habitat: A small perennial plant found in dry woods in Canada and USA.
Preparation: Tincture from entire fresh plant.

The medicine was introduced to Homeopathy by SA Jones (Pierce-377).

II. General Analysis (Cow.)

Acts markedly upon urinary apparatus, primarily upon bladder, then Kidneys. Very efficacious in catarrhal inflammation of urinary tract and bladder (Cystitis). Recommended in retention of urine, suppression of urine in infants (Acon.). Acute Prostatitis with retention of urine. Urine high coloured, offensive, turbid, with plenty of ropy or bloody mucous. Burning, scalding during urination, before and after, (Compare Acon., Apis., Apocy., Cann. sat., Canth., Equis.).

III. Clinical (Clarke-I-473)

Acne, Breast-atrophy of; cancer of; tumour of, Cataract, Cystitis, Diabetes, Dropsy, Fever, Glands enlarged, Gleet, Gonorrhoea, Intermittents, Jaundice, Kidney-affections of, Lactation disordered, Liver disorder, Nephritis, Proctitis, Prostatitis, Pterygium, Ringworm, Scrofula, Stricture, Syphilis, Toothache, Ulcers-malignant, Urinary disorders, Whitlow.

IV. **Symptoms-Particular** (Nash-421)

1. Cystitis-Ropy Mucous in urine: key symptom.
2. Sensation of swelling near anus in the perineum as if sitting on a ball.
   China +++
   Cann. ind. +

CHINA

I. Introduction (Cow.-248)

Synonym: Cinchona Officianalis, Cinchona Calisaya.
Natural Order: Rubiaceae.
Common Name: China, Yellow Peruvian Bark.
Habitat: A tall tree growing in Bolivia, Southern Peru.
Preparation: Tincture and Trituration from the powdered bark.

Hahnemann introduced this drug to Homeopathy in his MMP Vol. I Cinchona is to Homeopathy what falling apple was to Newton. In 1790 he first proved China on himself (1140 Symptoms) (Pierce-378).

II. General Analysis (Cow.)

Acts especially upon that portion of ganglionic (subsidiary nerve centre) nervous system which presides over vegetative functions, producing a condition of general depression and exhaustion, modifying the digestive functions. Blood circulation lacks energy, thus general debility, haemorrhage, profuse sweat, and urine, watery diarrhoea etc. It shows in vegetative sphere a great affinity for liver and spleen; in the former a long chain of biliary symptoms (Jaundice is one); in the later spleen enlargement. (Fever of malarial origin, periodicity being an essential feature). Chief characteristics are—excessive sensitiveness to touch, least contact, motion, physical or mental effort; prostration with neither thirst nor hunger.

III. Suited to (Allen-99)

Stout, Swarthy persons; once healthy now debilitated. 'Broken down' from exhausting discharges (Carb. v.). Apathetic, indifferent, taciturn (Phos. ac.), Despondent, gloomy, has no desire to live but lacks courage to commit suicide, Ailments from loss of fluids, esp. Haemorrhage.

IV. Clinical (Clarke-I-476)

Abscess, Alcoholism, Amblyopia, Anaemia, Aphthae, Apoplexy, Apoplexy, Appetite disordered Asthma, Back-weakness of, Bilious attack, Catarrhal affections, Coma, Constipation, Cough, Debility, Delirium, Diarrhoea, Dropsy, Dyspepsia, Ears-deafness; noises in, Emissions, Empyaema, Erysipelas, Facial neuralgia, Gall-stone colic, Haemorrhage, Haemorrhoids, Headache, Hectic fever, Hip-joint disease, Ichthyosis, Impotence, Influenza, Intermittent fever, Jaundice, Labour Lactation, Leucorrhoea, Lienteria, Liver-diseases of; cirrhosis of, Meniere's disease, Menstruation disordered, Mercury-effects of, Muscoe volitantes, Neuralgia, Peritonitis, Perspiration profuse, Pleurisy, Prosopoplagia, Psoriasis, Pylorus-disease of, Rheumatism, Self-abuse, Sleep disordered, Spermatorrhoea, Spleen-affections of, Suffocation-fits of, Taste disordered, Tea-effects of, Thirst, Tinnitus, Tobacco-habit, Traumatic fever, Tympanites, Veins-varicose, Vertigo.

V. Symptoms-General (Nash-46-47)

1. Debility and other complaints after excessive loss of fluids, blood letting etc.
2. Haemorrhage profuse, with faintness, loss of sight, ringing in the ears.
3. Great flatulence, with sensation as if the abdomen were packed full, not > by eructation of passing flatus. Painless diarrhoea (Yellow, watery), brownish, undigested.
4. Periodical affections especially every other day.
5. Excessive sensitiveness, especially to light touch, draft of air, hard pressure relieves.
6. Modalities-< from slight touch, least draft or air every other day, > by hard pressure on painful part.
7. Dropsy, following excessive loss of fluids; great debility, trembling, aversion to exercise; nervous, sensitive to touch, to pain, to drafts of air; unrefreshing sleep after 3 AM.

8. Face pale, Hippocratic; eyes sunken and surrounded by blue margins; pale, sickly expression, as after excesses.
9. Haemorrhage, from all outlets (Crotal. h., Sul. ac., Ferr.). Blood dark and clotted, with ringing in the ears, loss of sight, general coldness and sometimes Convulsion (Ferr. phos.).
10. General shaking chill over whole body.
11. Sweat, with great thirst; sweating during sleep, on being covered.

VI. Symptoms-Particular (Nash-47-52)

1. Great weakness, debility and other complaints after loss of fluids. Faintness, loss of sight, ringing in ears. Pale face, Throbbing headaches, sweats easily, Dark rings around eyes.
2. Great Flatulence, wish to belch up, but not relieved at all

   Carb. v.-Upper abdomen

   Lyc. -Lower abdomen

   China—Whole abdomen, so full and oppressed, can hardly breathe, and still hungry at meal time.
3. Stools-watery, undigested, painless. Large discharge of flatus(Calc. phos.).
4. Periodic affections—

   China -worse every other day

   Eup. perf. -worse cold, wet weather

   Ipec. -worse winter, dry weather

   Nat. m. -worse 10-11 AM

   Ars. -worse 1-2 AM/PM

   Nux. v. -worse 4 AM
5. Malaria (Intermittent Fever).

   China,

   Eup. perf.,

   Ign.,

   Caps.
6. Quinine Disorders—

   Ipec.,

   Puls.,

   Ars.,

Nat. m.,
Ferr.,
Nit. ac.,
Hep. s.,
Kali hydro.

7. Chronic Liver Troubles.
   Right-sided
8. Bleeding (Haemorrhage) from every outlet.
   China,
   Carb. v.,
   Ferr.,
   Crotal. h.,
   Phos.,
   Sul. ac.
9. Extreme sensitiveness to touch hard pressure (better).
   China-Hair-Blowing air on part.
   Asa.,
   Hep. s.,
   Lach.,
   Plumb.,
   Caps.—can hardly be shaved.

CICUTA VIROSA

I. Introduction (Cow.-238)

Natural Order: Umbelliferae.
Common Name: Water Hemlock, Cow Bane.
Habitat: Perennial plant near streams and ponds on wet lands in Germany and W. France.
Preparation: Tincture from the fresh root.

It was proved by Hahnemann (MMP 240 Symptoms) (Pierce-389).

II. General Analysis (Cow.)

Acts preeminently as a cerebrospinal irritant, producing tetanus, epileptic form of convulsion, local tonic and clonic (series of intermittent muscular contraction and relaxation) tonic (opp. of clonic). It resembles Nux. v. but difference is that in Nux. v. consciousness is not impaired, while in Cic. v. there is entire loss of consciousness.

III. Suited to (Allen-97)

Women subject to epileptic and choreic convulsion, spasm of teething children, or from worms, convulsion violent with distortion of body, renewed from touch, jar or noise puerperal convulsion. When reading letters go up or down or disappear (Cocc.). During dentition grinding of teeth.

IV. Clinical (Clarke-I-512)

Bladder-paralysis of, Cancer, Catalepsy, Cerebro-spinal meningitis, Coccygodynia, Concussions, Convulsions, Eczema, Epilepsy, Epithelioma, Eyes inflamed, Face-eruption on, Hiccough, Hysteria, Impetigo, Meningitis, Myelitis, Numbness, Oesophagus-constriction of, Paralysis, Psoriasis, Puerperal convulsions, Screaming, Strabismus,

Stuttering, Tetanus, Trismus, Waking-weeping on, Worm complaints.

V. **Symptoms-Particular** (Nash-267)

1. Excessively violent convulsion, odd shapes, and violent contortions After Cina. and after Arn., in convulsion.
2. Dentition-worms, after Cina. fails. Convulsion, concussion after Arn. fails.
3. Eczema-pustulates run together, yellow, thick scales on face and head etc.

VI. **Black Letter Symptoms** (Tyler-262)

- Absence of thought, difficulty of recollecting himself, deprivation of the senses.
- Anxiety; violently affected by sad stories.
- Moaning, whining and howling.
- Tranquillity of mind, he was extremely satisfied with his position and with himself, and very cheerful (curative secondary effect).
- Likes childish toys: jumps from bed in a happy, childish state.
- Very violent in all his actions.
- Anxious thoughts of the future: feels sad.
- Anxiety: excessively affected by sad stories.
- Mistrust and shunning of men: despises others.
- Vertigo: staggering.
- Pressive, stupefying headache, externally of forehead, more when at rest.
- Concussion of brain and chronic effects therefrom, especially spasms.
- Head bent backwards with Convulsion.
- Violent shocks through head, arms and legs, which cause them to jerk suddenly: head hot.
- Pupils first contracted, then very dilated.
- Dilated and insensible.
- Convergent strabismus in children, if periodic or spasmodic, or caused by Convulsion-blow or fall.
- Convulsion of facial muscles; distortions either horrible or ridiculous.

- Lockjaw.
- After swallowing a sharp piece of bone, or other injuries to oesophagus the throat closes, and there is danger of suffocation.
- Inability to swallow.
- Hiccough.
- Burning pressure in stomach, and abdomen.
- Throbbing in pit of stomach, which is swollen as large as a fist.
- Sudden shock in pit of stomach which causes opisthotonos.
- Distension and painfulness of abdomen.
- Colic with convulsion and vomiting.
- Frequent call to urinate.
- Trembling palpitation of heart.
- Feels as if heart stopped beating; sometimes faint feeling therewith.
- Tension or cramp in muscles of neck; if he turns head, can't easily turn it back again.
- Pain in nape, spasmodic drawing of head backward: with tremor of hand.
- The back bent backwards like an arch.
- Painful sensation on inner surface of scapula.
- Complete powerlessness of limbs, after spasmodic jerks.
- Frequent involuntary jerks and stitches in arms and fingers.
- A red vesicle on right scapula, very painful when touched.
- General convulsion. Epilepsy.
- Frightful epilepsy.
- Frightful distortion of the limbs and whole body.
- Convulsion with wonderful distortion of Limbs head turned backwards, back bent as in opisthotonos.
- Frightful convulsion.
- Epileptic fits, with swelling of stomach, as from violent spasm of the diaphragm. Hiccough; screaming; redness of face; trismus.
- Loss of consciousness, and distortion of limbs.

- Tonic spasm renewed from slightest touch; opening door, loud talking.
- An elevated eruption over whole face (and on both hands, as big as peas) which causes a burning pain when touched.
- Vivid dreams about events of day.
- Vivid unremembered dreams.
- Frequent waking out of sleep, in which he perspired all over, but from which he felt strengthened.
- They all wish to come near the warm stove.

CIMICIFUGA

I. Introduction (Cow.-241)

Synonym: Actea Racemosa. Macrotys.
Natural Order: Ranunculaceae.
Common Name: Black Cohosh, Black Snake Root, Rattle weed, squaw root.
Habitat: A perennial plant in the USA.
Preparation: Tincture from the fresh roots.

It was perhaps first proved by Dr. Hompel in about 1856 (Pierce-392).

II. General Analysis (Cow.)

It produces a depressing irritant condition under its effect on nervous system-irritation, inflammation, rheumatism and neuralgia with muscular spasm etc. and in Female generative organs, giving rise to various disorders indicating rheumatic and neuralgic disturbances of these parts. It resembles Bell., though less intense in its action upon brain-congestion, dilated pupils, vertigo etc.

III. Suited to (Allen-17)

See Actea Recemora.

IV. Clinical (Clarke-I-25)

Abortion-tendency to, Angina pectoris, Appetite disordered, Back pains, Breasts-affection of, Cerebro-spinal meningitis, Change of life, Chest-pains in, Chorea, Delirium tremens, Diaphragm-rheumatism of, Dyspepsia, Epilepsy. Faintness, Headache, Heart affections, Hyperpyrexia, Hypochondriasis, Hysteria, Lumbago, Melancholia, Meningitis, Menstruation disordered, Myalgia, Neuralgia, Ovaries-affections of, Perichondritis, Pleurodynia, Pregnancy-affections of, Puerperal mania, Rheumatic gout, Rheumatism, Sciatica, Side pain,

Sinking sensation, Sleeplessness, Spinal irritation, Stiff-neck, Tinnitus aurium, Tremors, Uterine affections, Vomiting of pregnancy.

V. **Black Letter Symptoms** (Tyler-272)

- Thinks she is going crazy.
- Mania following disappearance of neuralgia.
- Puerperal Mania.
- Incessant talking, changing from one subject to another.
- Feels grieved and troubles, with sighing: next day a feeling of tremulous joy, with mirthfulness, playfulness and clear intellect.
- Fear of death.
- Fullness and aching in vertex.
- Severe pains right side of Head, back of orbit.
- Brain as if too large; presses from within outwards.
- Dull constant, pain, especially occiput, extending to vertex.
- A pressing upwards and outwards, as if not room enough in upper portion of cerebrum; this pain was very oppressive and almost intolerable. A sense of soreness in occipital region, worse motion.
- Nausea. Retching, dilated pupils, tremor of limbs.
- Aching pain in both eyeballs.
- Sharp pain across hypogastrium.
- Abdominal muscles sore.
- Pains in uterine region, dart from side to side.
- Menses irregular, delayed or suppressed, with chorea, hysteria, or mental disease.
- Shivers, off first stage of labour.
- Infra-mammary pains, worse left side.
- Night cough, dry, incessant, short.
- Head and neck retracted.
- Rheumatic pains in muscle of neck and back ; feeling of stiffness.
- A severe drawing, tensive pain at the points of the spinous processes of the three upper dorsal vertebrae.
- Excessive muscular soreness.
- Rheumatic persons.

CINA

I. Introduction (Cow.-245)

Synonym: Artemesia Cina.
Natural Order: Compositae.
Common Name: Worm Seed.
Habitat: A native plant of the East, Persia and Asia Minor.
Preparation: Tincture from dried unexpanded flowers.

It was proved first by Hahnemann (Pierce-397).

II. General Analysis (Cow.)

Acts primarily upon intestinal canal producing symptoms indicating chronic irritation, inflammation and presence of intestinal worms. Its secondary action is upon brain and other organs.

III. Suited to (Allen-98)

Children with dark hair, very cross, irritable, ill-humoured, want to be carried, averse to caresses, desire many things but reject when offered (Ant. tar., Bry., Cham., Staph.). Constantly digging and boring at nose, itching of nose, rubs nose on pillow or shoulder of mother (Mar.). Child suffering from worms. Starts and screams, during sleep, grinds teeth (Cic. v., Spig.) Ascarides (worm in intestine) (Mar. v) Face is pale, sickly white and bluish appearance around mouth, one cheek red and other pale (Cham.).

IV. Clinical (Clarke-I-520)

Abdomen distended, Anaemia, Anus-irritation of, Asthenopia, Asthma, Bronchitis, Borborygmi, Chorea, Colic, Convulsions, Cough, Dentition, Diarrhoea, Enuresis, Eye affections, Hydrocephaloid, Intermittent fever, Leucorrhoea, Neuralgia, Remittent fever, Scarlatina, Sight-affections of, Spasms, Strabismus, Twitching, Urine milky, Whooping-cough, Worms.

V. Symptoms-General (Nash-357)

1. The child is cross and ugly, kicks and strikes; wants to be carried or rocked or don't want to be touched or looked at; wants things and pushed them away which offered.
2. Frequent boring the nose with the fingers.
3. Pale sickly look about the eyes, or white and blue about the mouth.
4. Frequent swallowing as if something came up in the throat.
5. Alternate canine hunger or no appetite at all.
6. Urine turns milky on standing.
7. Frequent sudden attacks of very high fever with glowing red hot face, with paleness around mouth and lips or sometimes alternates with dark bluish ring around the eyes.

VI. Symptoms-Particular (Nash-357)

Better results in 200 or higher potency.

1. Restless child at night due to worms; Screams out sharply in his sleep.

Apis. —Screams in sleep.
Cham. —Cross, wants to be carried.
Ant. c. —Does not want to be looked at, or carried.
Bry. } Staph. } Demands a thing then refuses when offered.
Cina —Face alternates with red hot face and pale sickly face.
Cham —Face one side red hot other pale and cold.

VII. Black Letter Symptoms (Tyler-282)

- Child exceedingly cross, cries and strikes at all around.
- Pitiful weeping, when awake.
- Can't be quieted by any persuasions; proof against

all caresses.

- Children wake in evening or before midnight with fear or fright, jump up, see sights, scream. Tremble and talk about it with much anxiety.
- When walking in open air stupefying, internal Headache, especially in sinciput, afterwards also occiput.
- Dull headache, effecting the eyes, in the morning.
- Looks sickly about the eyes, with paleness of face.
- Optical illusions in muscles of eyebrows, a kind of spasm.
- In external Ear, cramp-like twitchings.
- Dull stitches-a pinching pressure under the mastoid.
- Child frequently bores into nose till blood comes.
- Itching of nose. Child picks its nose very much, is very restless. Cries and is very inamiable.
- FACE pale and cold.
- White and blue about mouth.
- Burning heat over all face, rising heat and redness of cheeks without thirst after sleep.
- Adherent mucous in Larynx, in AM on rising; must often hawk.
- Great hunger soon after a meal: feeling of emptiness.
- Desires many and different things.
- Gnawing sensation in stomach, as from hunger.
- Very short breath, with interruptions: some inspirations are omitted.
- A kind of oppression of chest: the sternum seems to press on the lungs, and breathing is somewhat impeded.
- Hoarse hacking cough consisting of a few impulses, with long pauses before exciting irritation recurs; in the evening.
- Before coughing child raises herself suddenly, looks, wildly about: the body becomes stiff. She loses consciousness, as if she would have an epileptic spasm, then follows the cough.
- After coughing the child cries out, and a noise like gurgling is heard going down.
- Back and Limbs. Bruised pain in sacrum, not worse by movement.
- Drawing, tearing pain downwards through whole

spine.

- Boring. Cramping pain in left upper arm.
- Single, small, twitching stitches, in right, or left hand.
- Paralytic pain left thigh, not far from knee.
- Obtuse stitches here and there in the body.
- In body, limbs, arms, feet, toes, sometimes in the side, or on the back, or in nasal bones, but especially on the hip, obtuse stitches or squeezing or aching, or like knocks or jerks; on pressing the part if pains, as if sore or bruised.
- Convulsion of extensor muscles; child becomes suddenly stiff: there is a clucking noise, as though water were poured out of a bottle from throat down to abdomen.
- Worm spasms, the child stiffens out straight.
- When yawning, trembling of the body with shuddering.

CLEMATIS

I. Introduction (Cow-259)

Synonym: Clematis Erecta.
Natural Order: Ranunculaceae.
Common Name: Upright Virgin's Bower.
Habitat: A native plant of southern Europe.
Preparation: Tincture from the fresh roots and stems.

It was proved by Hahnemann. (Pierce-398)

II. General Analysis (Cow.)

Acts upon the skin, lymphatic (colourless fluid) glandular system, and the genito urinary organs.

III. Clinical (Clarke-I-533)

Cancer, Eye affections, Face-pimples on, Gonorrhoea, Headache, Rheumatism, Testicles inflamed, Toothache, Urethra-stricture of.

IV. Symptoms-Particular (Nash-440)

1. Stricture (Urethra) beginning of, gonorrhoeal, indicated by slow or intermittent out flow of urine. If given early it prevents stricture often (high).
2. Orchitis (Inflammation of testes) Testicles hard and swollen.

    Clem.—follows well Puls. (Puls.-Gonorrhoea suppressed).
    Puls.
3. Toothache

    Clem. } Better when cold water held in mouth.
    Coff. }

COCCULUS

I. Introduction (Cow.-263)

Synonym: Cocculus Indicus.
Natural Order: Menispermaceae.
Common Name: Indian Cockle, Indian Berries.
Habitat: A climbing shrub in Indian Peninsula.
Preparation: Tincture from coarsely powered dried fruit.

Hahnemann says that he was first to use it for medicinal use (555 symptoms) (Pierce-402).

II. General Analysis (Cow.)

Produces paralysis, tectonic convulsion, vertigo and confusion under its action upon nervous system and sensorium. It can cause symptom of sea sickness-nausea and faintness, weakness with vertigo which is its chief characteristic.

III. Suited to (Allen-102)

Women and children who suffer during menses and pregnancy, Unmarried and childless women, book worms, sensitive, romantic girls with irregular menses, Persons weak by sexual excess, Nausea-in carriage (Arn., Nux. m.) sea sick, carsickness, even at looking at a moving boat. Headache-in nape and occiput-spine as if tied by cord. Drunkard's diseases. Metallic taste, (Merc. c.) loss of appetite.

Time passes-too quickly. Too slowly (Arg. n., Cann. ind.). Weakness-It requires exertion to stand firmly, feels weak to talk, loss of sleep. Leucorrhoea-in place of menses or between periods (Lod., Xanth.), like washing of meat, easily offended, speaks hastily-Apis.). Vertigo, as if intoxicated when rising from bed. During Menses-too weak to stand due to weakness of lower Parts (Alumen, Carb. a).

IV. Clinical (Clarke-I-544)

Anger-effects of, Bone affections, Cerebro-spinal meningitis, Chorea, Colic, Convulsions, Debility, Faintness, Fear-effects of, Haemorrhoids, Headache, Hernia, Intermittent fever, Knee-weakness of; cracking in, Memory weak, Mental excitement-effects of, Menstrual headache, Menstruation painful, Overstrain-bodily or mental, Palpitation, Paralysis, Parotitis, Phthiriasis, Rheumatism, Riding in carriage-effects of, Sea-sickness, Sleep-affections from loss of, Somnolence, Spasms, Spinal irritation, Tympany, Vertigo, Vomiting.

V. Symptoms-General (Nash-170)

1. Weakness of cervical muscles, can hardly hold the head up.
2. Weakness in small of back as if paralysed, gives out when walking; can hardly stand, walk or talk.
3. Hands and feat get numb; asleep.
4. Headache with nausea and vomiting, gets faint and sick on rising up or riding in carriage or beat.
5. General sensation of weakness; or weak, hollow, gone feeling in head, stomach, abdomen etc. < by loss of sleep or night watching.
6. Great distension with flatulent colic, wind or menstrual colic; cramy pains, inclined to hernia.
7. Modalities; < sitting up, moving, riding in carriage or boat, smoking, talking, eating, drinking, night watching > when lying quite.

VI. Symptoms-Particular (Nash-170-75)

1. Prostration of nervous system.
2. Cerebro spinal system, can't hold head up; Back gives out when walking, Debility and Numbness, Paralytic pain in small of the back; Abdomen, Prostration, Depression.
3. < Sitting up, motion carriage, night watching (Nux. v.).
4. Hands and feet asleep at one time or another or first

one then another separately. Knees give out when walking, soles of feet as if asleep.

5. Dunham says that its sphere of action is pre-eminently the system of animal life; the voluntary muscular system first, and then the sensoriun are the primary seats of action. Nausea to the extent of vomiting, accompanied by serious faintness and vertigo when lifting the head, is characteristic of this medicine.
6. "It acts on voluntary muscles rather on intellectual power" (Pareira-171).
7. "Paralytic pain in the small of the back with spasmodic drawing of across the peeps, which prevents walking".
8. "His knees sink down from weakness, he totters while walking and threatens to fall to one side."
9. "At one time his feet are asleep, at another the hands."
10. "Hands tremble while eating, and the more the higher the hand is taken".
11. Soles of feet go to sleep white sitting.
12. This is picture of general prostration and spinal trouble coupled with following characteristic symptoms:

    ✓ Vertigo as if intoxicated and confusion of mind whirring vertigo while rising in bed, which compels to be down again.

    ✓ Sick headache with nausea with inclination to vomit (All these symptoms are < by riding in a carriage or boat).

    ✓ Sea sickness (sea sickness on deck in fresh cold air).

    ✓ Headache of Cocc. and Bry.

    ✓ Both < on rising up in the bed.

    Bry.-sickness in the stomach precedes headache.

    Cocc.-Reverse of Bry.

    ✓ Headache and vertigo.

    ✓ Accompanied with painful sensation of

weakness emptiness in the head; and in all internal parts.

Nausea with headache-persistent with aversion to food (in Colch.-more pronounced).

13. Metallic taste in the mouth.
14. Abdominal and uterine regions-great distension of the abdomen, focused in both flatulent colic and dysmenorrhea. In flatulent colic-sensation as if abdomen was full of. sticks or stones. Attacks of colic-at about midnight. Passing of flatus does not relieve much-forms again. In Dysmenorrhea-gripping and cramping pains, very severe with great weakness-can't stand or talk. (Carb. a..—great weakness but with flow, while in Coccu it is general and may not be related with flow)
15. Weak-Head cervical muscles-unable to support the head.

    Cocc.,

    Calc. phos.,

    Verat.
16. Vertigo-as Intoxicated, confusion of mind.
17. Whirling while rising up. Sick headache sick with nausea.

    Bry.-Stomach trouble leads than head.

    Calc. c.-Head first stomach later.
18. Abdomen distended as if with stones or sticks.

    Carb. a.-Mensrual flow weakness with.
19. < Carriage Riding (Nit. ac. better).
20. Emptiness in various organs.

VII. Black Letter Symptoms

(Tyler-295-98)

- Thoughts are fixed on a single disagreeable subject, absorbed in thought and notices nothing about her.
- Sits in deep reverie.
- Ill effects of anger and grief.
- Sudden extreme anxiety.
- Easily startled.

- Time passes too quickly.
- Stupid in the Head.
- Cloudiness of the head, chiefly after eating and drinking.
- Vertigo as if intoxicated, with dullness in forehead: as if a board across head: on rising from lying, had to tie down again.
- Vertigo: as if intoxicated with confusion: with nausea: things whirl from right to left.
- With flushed, hot face and head: then palpitation.
- Headache as if eyes would be torn out.
- Headache with nausea and inclination to vomit.
- Sick headache from riding in carriage, boat, train, cars, etc.
- Seasickness.
- Dimness of Sight.
- Dryness of oesophagus.
- Loss of appetite with metallic taste.
- Unusual Nausea and inclination to vomit, while riding in a wagon.
- Extreme aversion to food, caused even by the smell of food, although with hunger.
- Frequent empty Eructation.
- When he becomes cold, or catches cold, there is inclination to vomit, causing a copious flow of saliva.
- Inclination to vomit in connection with headache, and a pain as if bruised in the bowels.
- Violent spasm in the Stomach, clutching in the stomach.
- Spasm in the stomach: squeezing in the stomach.
- Griping in epigastrium, taking away the breath.
- Thirst especially for beer.
- Great distension of the Abdomen.
- Flatulent colic about midnight; awakened by incessant accumulation of flatulence, which distended the abdomen, causing oppressive pain here and there; some was passed without remarkable relief, whilst new flatus constantly collected for several hours; he was obliged to lie on one side for relief.
- Painful inclination to a hernia, especially after rising from sitting.

- Watery urine.
- Itching in scrotum.
- Menstruation seven days too early, with distension of abdomen and cutting, contracting pains in abdomen on every motion and every breath, together with contraction of rectum.
- Tensive construction of right side Chest, which oppresses the breathing.
- Very violent tickling in larynx, wakes him at 11. 30 PM, causes cough, with expectoration of much tenacious mucous.
- Expectoration of much viscid albuminous mucous.
- Paralytic Symptoms.
- Weakness of cervical muscles, with heaviness of head.
- In shoulder joint and muscles of upper arm, single stitches when at rest.
- Stitches in right upper arm.
- Numbness and paralytic feelings in arms.
- Now one hand, now the other is numb, as if asleep.
- Sometimes one hand, sometimes the other is alternately hot and cold.
- Hand trembles while eating, and the more the higher it is raised.
- Knees sink down from weakness; totters while walking and threatens to fall to one side.
- Cracking of the knee when moving.
- Soles of both feet go to sleep while sitting.
- At one time the feet are asleep, at another the hands, (And, in italics weakness in limbs as if paralysed.)
- Trembling from excitement, over-exertion and pain.
- Sensation of seasickness.
- Hysteric complaints with sadness.
- Convulsion after loss of sleep.
- Attacks of paralytic weakness with pain in back.
- Here and there in the limbs an acute paralytic drawing, continuous and in jerks, as if in the bone.
- Cracking and creaking in the joints.
- Painful stiffness of the joints.
- Falling asleep of feet and hands alternately, in short paroxysms.

- Tendency to tremble.
- Great exhaustion of the body, so that it was an exertion to him to stand steady.
- Slight perspiration over the whole body on slightest exertion.
- Cocc. excites shooting pains and heat in cold glandular swelling, at least when they are touched.
- All the symptoms and sufferings, especially in the head, are aggravated by drinking, eating, sleeping and speaking.
- Intolerance of cold and warm air.
- Sleep disturbed by excessive anxiety and restlessness.
- Sleepless from long continued nursing; from night watching.
- Anxious, frightful dreams.
- Ill effects from loss of sleep and night watching.
- *Fever Symptoms.*
- Chill frequently alternating with heat.
- Flushes of heat, with burning heat of cheeks and cold feet.
- Insidious nervous Fever, particularly in cases which have been produced by frequent fits of anger, or are accompanied by great disposition to anger.

COFFEA CRUDA

I. Introduction (Cow.-272)

Synonym: Coffea Arabica.
Natural Order: Rubiaceae.
Common Name: Coffee.
Preparation: Tincture from un-roasted coffee beans.
It was proved by Hahnemman (Pierce-407).

II. General Analysis (Cow.)

Acts upon cerebro spinal nervous system, producing excitation of special senses, acute sensitiveness, Chief characteristics are excitation of special senses, great sensitiveness to pain, sleeplessness from excitement.

III. Suited to (Allen-104)

Tall, lean, stooping persons, sanguine, choleric temperament (hasty, prone to emotional out bursts) over sensitiveness of all senses(Bell., Cham., Op.) Bad effect of sudden emotions or pleasant surprises Pain felt insupportable (Acon., Cham.), Hasty eating and drinking. Headache-from mental exertion, one sided as if a nail driven into brain (Ign., Nux. v.).

IV. Clinical (Clarke-I-556)

Apoplexy, Asthma, Aural neuralgia, Colic, Convulsions, Diarrhoea, Ecstasy, Excitement, Headache, Heart-hyperaesthesia of, Hernia, Hyperaesthesia, Hysteria, Intermittents, Joy-ill effects of, Labour pains, Metrorrhagia, Neuralgia, Over-sensitiveness, Sciatica, Shock, Sleeplessness, Toothache.

V. Symptoms-General (Nash-161)

1. All senses more acute; reads fine print easier, smell,

taste and touch acute, unusual activity of mind and body, full of ideas, quick to act, no sleep on this account, etc.

2. Affections from sudden surprises, especially joyful surprises, very emotional.
3. Pains insupportable, drive to despair; exasperation, tears, tossing about in agony; great sleeplessness.
4. Headache, from over mental exertion, thinking, talking; one-sided, as from a nail driven into the brain (Ign., Nux. v.); as if the brain were torn or dashed to pieces < in open air.
5. Jarring toothache; relieved by holding ice water in the mouth; returns when water becomes warm.

VI. Symptoms-Particular (Nash 162-3)

1. Acts strongly upon nervous system like Cham.
2. Mental. Like Cham. but mind of Cham. is not there.
3. Acon.—fear of death but in Cham. it is not there.
4. Herring used to alternate Acon. and Coff. in painful inflammatory affections with fever where fever symptoms of Acon. and nervous sensibility of Coff. were present. Coff.—especially adopted to mental shock such as sudden surprises, excessive laughter etc., disappointed love, strong smells etc.
5. Pain Remedy.

   Acon.,

   Cham.—Pain of coffee drinker especially.

   Coff.—Pains of coffee drinkers do not suit it. Pains insupportable, drive to despair, tears tossing about in great anguish.
6. One sided Headache.

   Coff. —As if nail driven in to the head (Ign.).

   Ign. —as if hysterical.
7. Toothache (Prosopoplagia).

   Cham. < hot things but not better by cold things as in Coff.

   Coff. > cold as long remains cold in mouth.
8. Dysmenorrhoea with excessive painful colic.

   Coff. —large clots (intolerable pains, with no especially leading symptoms.).

Cham. —if Coff. does not relieve then Cham.

9. Sleeplessness.

Coff. —from activity of mind. (better 200 potency).

Cham. —from sensitiveness.

VII. Black Letter Symptoms (Tyler-300-1)

- Unusual activity of mind and body.
- Full of ideas; quick to act, no sleep on this account.
- Mental excitability.
- Sleeplessness on account of excessive mental and physical excitement.
- Fright from sudden pleasant surprises.
- Pains seem in-supportable driving to despair.
- Affections after sudden emotions, particularly pleasant surprises.
- All the senses more acute, reads fine print easier, particularly an increased perception of slight passive motions.
- Threatening of apoplexy; over-excited, talkative, full of tear, pangs of conscience, aversion to open air.
- Sleepless, convulsive grinding of teeth.
- One-sided headache, as from a nail driven into head (Thuj..); worse in open air.
- Neuralgic toothache entirely relieved by holding cold water in the mouth, returning as this becomes warm.
- During labour or after pain extreme fear of death.
- Great agitation and restlessness.
- Affections after sudden emotions, especially pleasant surprises.
- Would like to rub or scratch the part, but it is too sensitive.
- Bad effects from wine or liquor drinking.
- Thirst at night wakes him during sweat, infrequent during heat; almost constant thirst after heat and during sweat.

COLCHICUM AUTUMNALE

I. Introduction (Cow.-274)

Synonym: Colchicum Autumnale.
Natural Order: Melanthaceae.
Common Name: Meadow saffron.
Habitat: Perennial plant growing in meadows in Germany, France and South Europe.
Preparation: Tincture from the fresh bulbs, before blooming.

It was first proved by Staff, one of Hahnemann's provers (Pierce-409).

II. General Analysis (Cow.)

Acts upon cerebrospinal and ganglionic nervous system producing cramp, convulsion, debility etc. Its more important action is upon periosetum, synovial membranes (of small joints) upon urinary and digestive tract. Violent, acute, arthritic inflammation. Gout, Chief peculiarity is its tearing pain with intolerable exacerbation at night.

III. Suited to (Allen-105)

Rheumatic, gouty-diathesis, robust vigorous constitution, diseases of old age. Smell painfully acute, nausea and faintness from cooking odours. Bad effects of night watching (Cocc.).

IV. Clinical (Clarke-I-563)

Appendicitis, Asthma, Cataract, Cholera, Colic, Cough, Cramps, Debility, Diabetes, Diarrhoea, Dropsy, Dysentery, Eye affections, Feet-pain in, Gout, Heart affections, Ileus, Intermittent fever, Intestinal catarrh, Lumbago, Myalgia, Nephritis (rheumatic and gouty), Pericarditis, Proctalgia, Prostatitis, Rectum-prolapse of, Rheumatism, Stiff-neck, Tongue-sensibility lost, Typhlitis, Typhoid fever.

V. **Symptoms-General** (Nash-406)

1. The smell of food nauseates to faintness.
2. Fall dysenteries, when days are warm and nights are cool; stools shreddy and bloody, like scrappings.
3. Swelling of joints moving from one place to another, they are often dropsical, and pit on pressive < in extremeness of wet and cold or warm and dry (Kent).

VI. **Symptoms-Particular** (Nash-406)

1. Sundown to Sunrise-all symptoms worse.
2. Smell of cooking nauseates to faintness. Colch.—key symptom.
3. Violent burning pains and icy coldness in the stomach. These opposites are found in the stomach.
4. Stools-shreddy bloody scrapping like, as if mucous membrane.
   Canth.,
   Colch.,
   Carb. v.,
   China,
   Lyc.
5. Dyspepsia with complaint of burning or coldness (icy) in the stomach and much gas in stomach or abdomen or both. Colc. some times takes precedence over Lyc., China, Carb. v.
6. Appendicitis-with Colc. Symptom.

VII. **Black Letter Symptoms** (Tyler-307-9)

- Memory weakened, ideas not so clear as usual: forgetfulness, absence of mind.
- External impressions, bright light, strong odours, contact, misdeeds of others, make him quite beside himself.
- Strong odours make him quite beside himself.
- Aversion to Food; loathing the sight, and still more the smell of it.
- No thirst.
- Smell of cooking nauseates to faintness.

- Nausea, Eructation and copious vomiting of mucous and bile.
- Violent retching followed by copious and forcible vomiting of food and then of bile.
- Violent burning in epigastrium.
- Very painful urging to Stool. Only a little faeces passed, then followed transparent, gelatinous, and very membranous mucous, with some relief of the pain in the abdomen.
- Extremely painful stools.
- Discharge from bowels like gelatine.
- Watery, jelly-like mucous passes from anus with violent spasm in sphincter.
- Bloody stools with scrapings from intestines and protrusion of anus.
- Autumn dysentery, with discharges of white mucous and violent tenesmus; bloody stools, mingled with a slimy substance.
- Bloody discharge from bowels with deathly nausea from smelling cooking.
- Tenesmus in rectum.
- Discharge from bowels containing a large quantity of small white shreddy particles.
- Pain in region of Kidneys.
- Urine like ink.
- Stinging and tearing in muscle of chest; pleurodynia.
- Oppression of chest, dyspnoea, a tensive feeling in chest, sometimes high, sometimes low down.
- Oppression of chest with violent palpitation.
- Hydrothorax with oedema of hands and feet.
- Pulse thread-like, imperceptible.
- Effusion into pericardium after inflammatory affections of heart.
- A paralytic pain in the arms, so violent he can't hold the lightest thing firmly.
- Lameness after suddenly checked sweat, particularly on feet by getting wet all over.
- At the beginning of acute rheumatism before fully developed.

- Pains in shoulder and hip-joints, and in all bones, with difficulty in moving head and tongue.
- Great weakness and exhaustion, as after exertion, can't move head from pillow.
- Fall dysentery.
- Constant chilly feeling, even when sitting near stove, with flushes of heat.
- Pain goes from left to right in gout.
- Rheumatic pains excited by or worse for cold damp weather.
- Acute dropsy with renal affections.
- Uric Acid diathesis.
- Gout in person of vigorous constitutions.

COLLINSONIA CANADENSIS

I. Introduction (Cow.-278)

Synonym: Collinsonia Canadensis.
Natural Order: Labiatae.
Common Name: Stone root, Horsebalmn, Rich weed.
Habitat: An indigenous plant, growing in rich moist woods of Canada to Florida, and west to Michigan.
Preparation: Tincture from the fresh root.

It was proved by Dr. WH Burt. (Pierce-413)

II. General Analysis (Cow.)

Acts predominantly upon gastrointestinal canal, especially rectum, affects in a marked degree the heart and the generative organs. Chief action-haemorrhoids caused by intertia and congestion of portal region, and related functional troubles arising therefrom.

III. Suited to (Allen-106)

Patients with piles and indigestion. Palpitation, Rapid heart action but weak. Chronic, painful bleeding piles, as if sand in rectum (Aesc. hip.). After heart is relieved, piles or menses (suppressed) return. Persons with alternate constipation with diarrhoea.

IV. Clinical (Clarke-I-568)

Constipation, Diarrhoea, Dropsy (cardiac), Dysentery, Dysmenorrhoea, Dyspepsia, Haemorrhage, Haemorrhoids, Heart affections, Irritation, Labour, Pregnancy-affections of, Proctitis, Pruritus vulvae, Rheumatism.

V. Symptoms-Particular (Nash-438)

1. Most obstinate constipation, Rectal Troubles.

Aesc. hip.	**Collin.**
Sense of fullness	No
Piles do not bleed	As a rule bleed
Pain in back	No
Sometimes constipated	Always constipated

VI. Black Letter Symptoms (Tyler-311)

- Mucous or black and faecal stools with colic and tenesmus (after confinement).
- Haemorrhoidal dysentery with tenesmus.
- Obstinate constipation with haemorrhoids, stools very sluggish and hard, accompanied by pain and flatulence.
- Piles with constipation, or even with diarrhoea, bleeding, or blind and protruding: feeling of sticks, gravel, or sand in rectum: evening and night: better in morning.
- Flowing piles, haemorrhoids incessant though not profuse, with alternative constipation and diarrhoea.
- Chronic, bleeding, painful haemorrhoids.
- Dropsy from cardiac disease.

COLOCYNTHIS

I. Introduction (Cow.-280)

Synonym: Cucumis Coloncynthis. Citrullus Coloncythis.
Natural Order: Cucurbitaceae.
Common Name: Squirting Cucumber, Bitter apple.
Habitat: A slender plant with perennial root growing in dry regions of Western Hemisphere.
Preparation: Tincture from dried fruit, freed from outer rind and seed.

Hahnemann proved it (MMP 250 symptoms) (Pierce-414).

II. General Analysis (Cow.)

Acts upon ganglionic nervous system produces neuralgia, irritation and inflammation. Profound action upon alimentary canal causing vomiting, purging and intense colic. Neuralgia of face, eyes, and head. Chief characteristics are—severe colicky pains, better by bending double and worse in any other position.

III. Suited to (Allen-107)

Extremely irritable, impatient, become angry or offended on being questioned. Affections from anger-Colic, vomiting, Diarrhoea and suppression of menses (Cham., Staph.). Agonizing pain in abdomen causing to bend double, > hard pressure (> heat Mag. phos.). < by bending double (Diosc.).

IV. Clinical (Clarke-I-572)

Cataract, Ciliary neuralgia, Colic, Coxalgia, Diabetes, Diarrhoea, Dysentery, Dysmenorrhoea, Glaucoma, Headache, Hoarseness, Menstrual colic, Neuralgia, Ovaries-affections of, Paraphimosis, Peritonitis, Rheumatism, Sciatica, Toothache, Tumours, Uterus-pains in, Vagina-Pains in.

V. **Symptoms-General** (Nash-392)

1. Disinclined to talk, to see friends; impatient, easily offended, anger with indignation; colic or other complaints as a consequence.
2. Colic, terrible; they seek relief by bending double or pressing sometimes hard against the abdomen.
3. Dysentery-like diarrhoea; renewed after least food or drink, often with the characteristic colic pains.
4. Frequent urging to urinate, scanty; urine sometimes thick, foetid, viscid, jelly-like.
5. Crampy pain in sciatica nerve, from hip down posterior portion of thigh; > from hard pressure and from heat; < in repose, driving patient desperate.
6. Tendency to painful Cramp, with all pains.
7. Modalities: < evening, anger; after eating; > from coffee; bending double and head pressure.

VI. **Symptoms-Particular** (Nash-393-396)

1. Colic-most severe-Crampy-Neuralgic, often attended with vomiting and diarrhoea, rather on account of great pain than any derangement of bowel, etc. Terrible Colic > double up.

   Mag. phos., Ars.—hot application with.

   Cham., Coloc.—much wind distending stomach; fit of anger brings Colic.

   Staph.—Child colic with teeth decay and black teeth; sore eyelids.

   Verat.—like Coloc. but with cold sweat and patient walks for relief.

   Bov., Coloc. > eating > by bending double like Coloc.

   Diosc.—wind colic from umbilical but unlike Coloc. which is > doubling up. Pain begins at umbilicus then radiates all over. (Plumb.-walls retracted)

   Jal. —Colic with diarrhoea, child cries day and night.

   Stan.—child's colic, abdomen on mother's shoulders.

2. Sciatica (Facial and Sciatic Neuralgia).
   (Mag. phos. = Coloc. in crampy Colic > heat).
   Coloc.—From hip to posterior portion of thigh (Bry. >lying on painful side).
   Bry.-> lying on painful side.
   Phyt.—pain runs down outer side of thigh.
   Gnaf., Bry., Coloc., Phyt. are leading remedies of this malady.

VII. Black Letter Symptoms
(Tyler-318-9)

- Pressing, aching pain in the sinciput, most violent on stooping and when lying on the back.
- Tearing pain in the whole brain, which became a pressure in the forehead, as if it pressed out the forehead-more violent on moving the eyelids.
- Burning pain in the skin of forehead above eyeball.
- Sharp, cutting pain in the right eyeball.
- Throbbing and digging pain from middle of the left side of nose, to the root of nose.
- Pain in lower row of teeth, as if the nerve were tugged and stretched.
- Empty Eructation.
- Constrictive pain in umbilicus, immediately after dinner.
- Seized with terrible, contractive, twisting pain in the bowels, immediately about umbilicus.
- Griping about umbilicus.
- Griping around the navel, increased by eating fruit.
- Griping and cutting in umbilical region.
- Violent griping in the umbilical region.
- Violent colic-like pains, emanating from the umbilicus, with frequent discharge of flatus, which afforded relief.
- Isolated deep stitches, as if from a needle, sometimes in the left, sometimes in the right flank, apparently connected with the ovaries.
- Abdomen greatly distended and painful.
- Griping in the abdomen, especially about the navel.
- Griping and pinching in abdomen.

- Violent griping pains in abdomen, worst about three fingers breadth below the navel, obliging him to bend over.
- Griping in the intestines as if the bowels would be forcibly griped.
- Pinching pain in the abdomen, as if the bowels were pressed inward, with cutting extending towards the pubic region, so severe below the naval that the muscles of the face are distorted and the eyes drawn together (Closed): the pain is only relieved by pressure upon the bowels with the hands and bending himself forward.
- Pinching in the bowels as if the intestines were squeezed between stones.
- Cutting in the abdomen.
- Colic very violent in paroxysms, obliging him to bend forward. Colic of the most violent character. Griping colic.
- Urging to urinate.
- (Heavy weight in lumbo-dorsal region with some increase of temperature and sensibility on the part affected). The origin of the trouble lay in the sacral region, corresponding to the plexus ischiadicus, thence it extended through the incisure ischiadica major towards the hip joint, down the posterior portion of the thigh into the fossa poplitea.
- Tensive shooting pain in the right loin only felt on inspiration and most violent when lying on the back.
- Short cough when smoking tobacco.
- Sore pain in left scapula, when at rest.
- In region of right scapula, an internal drawing sensation, as if the nerves and vessels were stretched.
- Severe drawing, sharp pain in the left cervical muscles, still more severe on movement.
- Violent drawing pains in the thumb of the right hand.
- Only when walking, pain in the right thigh, as if the psoas muscle that raises it were too short; on standing it ceased, but on walking it returned.
- Tearing pain in the sole of the right foot, most violent when at rest.

CONIUM MACULATUM

I. Introduction (Cow.-285)

Synonym: Conium Maculatum.
Natural Order: Umbelliferae.
Common Name: Poison Hemlock. Spotted Hemlock.
Habitat: A native plant of Europe but naturalised in Eastern part of USA.
Preparation: Tincture from fresh plant. It is known as a poison from ancient times. Socrates was given a cup of this poison.

It was proved homoeopathically by Hahnemann for the first time (375 Symptoms) (Pierce-417).

II. General Analysis (Cow.)

Acts upon motor nervous tracts, producing paralytic conditions. It benumbs the brain and causes vertigo, dilated pupils and even convulsion. It affects glandular system profoundly, causing alternation in glandular substance, scrofulous and cancerous affections, Diseases of old people is its main characteristic.

III. Suited to (Allen-108)

Old people, old maids during and after climacteric, strong persons with sedentary habits. Debility of old people, complaints caused by fall or blow, of rigid fibre, cancerous, persons with enlarged glands, indolent, indifferent, memory weak, morose, easily vexed. Can't tolerate contradiction; excitement causes depression. Alone-dreads, Stony hardness of mammae, testicles etc; after injury of glands (=Ast. r.). Breasts-sore and hard before and during Menses. Urine-great difficulty in voiding, prostatic or uterine affections, menses feeble, suppressed, too late, scanty with red rash on body which ceases with flow of (Dulc.) Leucorrhoea

10 days after menses (Bor., Bov.). Vertigo-when lying down or turning in bed.

IV. Clinical (Clarke-I-581)

Asthma, Bladder-inflammation of, Breast-affections of; painful, Bronchitis, Bruises, Cancer, Cataract, Chorea, Cough, Depression of spirits, Diphtheritic paralysis, Dysmenia (membranous), Erysipelas, Eye affections, Galactorrhoea, Herpes, Hypochondriasis, Jaundice, Liver enlarged, Melancholia, Menstruation disordered, Numbness, Ovaries-affections of, Paralysis; Landry's, Peritonitis, Phthisis, Pregnancy-painful breasts during, Prostatitis, Ptosis, Scrofula, Spermatorrhoea, Sterility, Stomach-affections of, Testicles-affections of, Tetters, Trismus, Tumours, Ulcer, Vertigo, Vision disordered, Wens.

V. Symptoms-General (Nash-175)

1. Vertigo, especially < on turning the head or looking around sidewise, or turning in bed.
2. Swelling and induration of glands, after contusions or bruises.
3. Cancerous and scrofulous persons with enlarged glands.
4. Urine flows, stops and flows again intermittently, prostatic or uterine affections.
5. Breasts sore, hard and painful during menstrual period.

VI. Symptoms-Particular (Nash-175-9)

1. Spinal remedy.
2. Vertigo on—
   a. Head turning on-(Con., Calc. c., Kali c..)
   b. While moving head-(Bry., Calc. c., Con.)
   c. From odour of flowers-(Nux. v., Phos.)
   d. While looking up-(Puls., Sil.)
   e. While looking down-(Phos., Spig., Sul.)
   f. From loss of sleep-(Nux. v., Cocc.)
   g. From least noise-(Ther.)

h. While walking-(Nat. m., Nux. v., Phos., Puls.)
i. While studying-(Nat. m.)
j. While eating or after-(Grat., Nux. v., Puls.)
k. As if whirling-(Bry., Con., Cycl., Puls.)
l. With fainting-(Nux. v.)
m. With staggering-(Arg. n., Gels., Nux. v., Phos.)
n. On eyes closed or in dark-(Arg. n., Stram., Ther.)
o. With dimness of sight-(Cycl., Gels., Nux. v.)
p. When rising from seat-(Bry., Phos.)
q. When rising from stooping-(Bell.)
r. When rising from bed-(Bry., Chel., Cocc.)
s. When stooping-(Bell., Nux. v., Sul., Puls.)
t. When Ascending-(Calc. c.)
u. When descending-(Bor., Ferr.)
v. When Lying-(Con.)
w. When must lie down-(Bry., Cocc., Phos., Puls.)
x. When Occipital-(Gels., Sil., Petr.)
y. When after sleep-(Lach.)
z. When after suppressed Menses-(Cycl., Puls.)

3. Eye-Photophobia (no tolerance of light), out of all proportions, to the objective signs of inflammation < Night, even ray of light, > pressure, dark room.
4. Falling of Eye lids.
   Con.,
   Gels.,
   Caust.,
   Sep.
5. Lump or swelling, results of blow or injury, cancerous or benign, of stony hardness. First remedy to be thought of in such symptoms.
   Carb. a.,
   Con.,
   Sil.,
   Ast. r. (Lacerating pain)
6. Sex (Male).
   Con.-intense desire but unable to perform
   Lyc.,
   Agar.,
7. Intermittent flow of urine.
   Acon.,
   Clem.,

Con.-Hypertrophy of the prostate gland incident to the old age. Sweat during sleep.

8. Strong Hardness of Mammae-Con. is remedy to be thought off.

   Con. -Right
   Sil. -left.
   Ast. r. -acute lancinating pains.

9. All scirrhous affections of the breast.

VII. Black Letter Symptoms (Tyler-327)

- Inability to sustain any mental efforts.
- Hypochondriasis and hysteria from suppression of or too free indulgence in sexual instinct, with low-spiritedness, anxiety and sadness.
- Want of Memory.
- Excessive difficulty to recollect things; to comprehend that which one reads.
- Headache as if head were too full and would burst.
- Sick headache with inability to urinate. Great giddiness, worse lying, when everything seems to go round.
- Vertigo as if turning in a circle.
- Intoxication when talking the least liquor.
- Accumulation of Ear-wax; blood red or like decayed paper with pus or mucous.
- Weakness of Sight; amaurosis.
- Objects look red, rainbow-coloured, striped; confused spots.
- Weakness and dazzling of eyes with giddiness and debility of whole body especially muscles of arms and legs, so that when I attempted to walk I was apt to stagger like a person who had drunk too much strong liquor.
- Aversion to light without inflammation of eyes.
- Burning in eyes.
- Ulcers on cornea, right to left.
- Could scarcely raise lids, they seemed pressed down with a heavy weight.

- Intermittent flow of Urine with cutting after micturition.
- Some sexual symptoms, Bad effects from suppressed desire, or excessive indulgence.
- Shrivelling of mammae, without sexual desire.
- Dry spot in larynx, where there is crawling and almost constant irritation to dry Cough.
- Cough, almost only when first lying down, during day or evening: obliged to sit up and cough it out, then had rest.
- Powerful spasmodic paroxysm of cough, excited by itching and tickling in chest and throat, or by a dry spot in larynx, worse at night or lying down, greatly fatiguing patient.
- Lying down and taking a deep breath causes cough.
- Stitches as with needless in left Mamma.
- Hardness of right breast, with painfulness to touch and nightly stitches in it.
- Pain in mamma, which often swell and become hard.
- Hard, scirrhus-like tumours (breast).
- Indurated and swollen cervical Glands in scrofulous children.
- Tremulous weakness and palpitation after every stool.
- Paroxysms of hysteria and hypochondriasis from abstinence from sexual intercourse.
- Great heat internal and external, with great nervousness.
- Sweat day and night, as soon as one sleeps, or even when closing eyes.
- Swelling and induration of glands, with tingling and stitches, after contusions and bruises.
- With all his efforts he could not keep off Sleep; must lie down and sleep; or he only gets sleep after midnight.

COPAIVA

I. Introduction (Clarke-I-592)

Synonym: Copaiva officinelis.
Natural Order: Leguminosae.
Preparation: Tincture of the balsam.

II. Clinical (Clarke-I-592)

Acne, Anus-itching of, Bladder irritable, Blenorrhagia, Bronchitis, Catarrh, Cough, Cystitis, Dysentery, Fistula, Gastritis, Gonorrhoea, Haemorrhoids, Measles, Nose-bleed, Prostatitis, Pruritus, Urethritis, Urticaria, Vulva-inflammation of.

III. Symptoms-Particular (Nash-441)

Acts upon Mucous Membrane

1. Chronic bronchial catarrh-profuse expectoration greenish purulent matter.
    - Cop.—disgusting smelling sputa.
    - Stan.,
    - Lyc.,
    - Sul.,
    - Phos.

    New Medicines
    - Yebra Santa,
    - Balsam,
    - Myosotis,
    - Pix liquida,
    - Illiciuma,
2. Urine—irritation in and at neck of urethra (valuable remedy in Gonorrhoea).
    - Cop. +
    - Canth. ++

CORALLIUM

I. Introduction (Cow-291)

Synonym: Corallium Rubram.
Natural Order: Gorgoniadeae.
Common Name: Red Coral.
Preparation: Triturations.

II. General Analysis (Cow.)

Acts upon respiratory tract causing catarrhal conditions giving rise to difficult breathing and profuse mucous accumulation.

III. Clinical (Clarke-I-594)

Asthma Milleri, Catarrh, Chancre, Cough, Eruptions, Glands inflamed, Hysteria, Measles, Post-nasal catarrh, Psoriasis, Purpura, Syphilis, Whooping-cough.

IV. Symptoms-Particular (Nash-439)

Useful for Spasmodic Cough.

1. Minute Gum cough < night, night paroxysm very serious.
2. Nose-catarrh with dropping in throat.
   Coral. r.,
   Nat. c.
3. Cancer: Ulcer red, exceedingly sensitive, painful.

CROCUS SATIVUS

I. Introduction (Cow.-292)

Synonym: Crocus Sativus.
Natural Order: Iridaceae.
Common Name: Saffron.
Habitat: A perennial native plant of Asia Minor, now cultivated in most temperate countries.
Preparation: Tincture from dried stigmas.

II. General Analysis (Cow.)

Acts upon cerebrospinal system producing brain irritation, congestion and hysterical mania. Passive uterine haemorrhage-blood dark, clotted and stringy are its chief characteristic.

III. Suited to (Allen-110)

Persons with frequent and extreme changes in sensations, Suddenly from greatest hilarity to deepest despondency (Ign., Nux. m). Haemorrhage from any part, every drop can be turned into a thread, hangs from the bleeding surface, Headache during climacteric, pulsating, throbbing; Nervous or menstrual headache, before, during, after the flow (Lach., Lil. t., Sec.).

IV. Clinical (Clarke-I-606)

Abortion threatened, After-pains, Anger, Asthenopia, Blepharospasm, Brain-congestion of, Chorea, Dysmenia, Fainting, Gastric disorders, Haemoptysis, Haemorrhage, Headache, Heart affections, Hysteria, Lachrymation, Laughter, Leucorrhoea, Mania, Menstruation-profuse, Metrorrhagia, Nose-bleed, Operation-effects of, Ophthalmia, Pregnancy-imaginary; Pregnancy-affections of, Tumours, Ulceration, Wounds.

V. **Symptoms-General** (Nash-410)

1. Spasmodic contractions and twitching of single sets of muscles.
2. Haemorrhage from different parts; blood black, viscid, clotted, forming into long black strings, from the bleeding orifice.
3. Changeable disposition; laughs, sings, jumps, wants to kiss everybody, or again cries, gets mad, abuses everybody, etc.
4. Sensation as of something hopping or moving about in stomach, abdomen, uterus or chest.

VI. **Symptoms-Particular** (Nash-410)

1. Haemorrhage from different parts-black viscid, in long black string.
   Croc. ++
   Merc. s. + Blood hangs from the nose like an icicle.
2. Hysterical condition with great changeableness of the symptoms.
   Acon.,
   Ign.,
   Nux. m.,
   Croc. ++
3. Sensation of something moving, hopping in abdomen, chest, etc., so the movement appears that she thinks she is in family way.
4. Twitching of single set of muscles.
   Croc.—in hysterical persons.
   Ign.,
   Zinc.

CROTALUS HORRIDUS

I. Introduction (Cow.-295)

Natural Order: Ophidia.
Common Name: Rattle snake.
Preparation: Venom is received on milk sugar and triturated.

It was first proved by Hoering and published in 1837 (Pierce-427).

II. General Analysis (Cow.)

Acts upon primarily like other serpent poison cerebro spinal nerve centres, producing decomposition of blood, destruction of blood fibrin, haemorrhage etc. Main characteristics-Yellow fever like characteristics.

III. Suited to (Allen-111)

Strumous, debilitated, haemorrhagic, broken down constitutions, during Zymotic diseases, tendency to blood boil or Carbuncles (Anthrac.), Haemorrhagic diathesis.

IV. Clinical (Clarke-I-613)

Amblyopia, Apoplexy, Appendicitis, Bilious fever, Boils, Cancers, Carbuncles, Cerebro-spinal meningitis, Chancre, Ciliary neuralgia, Convulsions, Delirium tremens, Dementia, Diphtheria, Dysmenorrhoea, Dyspepsia, Ear-discharge from, Ecchymosis, Epilepsy, Eye affections, Erysipelas, Face-eruption on; distortion of, Haematuria, Haemorrhagic diathesis, Headache, Heart affections, Herpes, Hydrophobia, Intestinal haemorrhage, Jaundice, Keratitis, Liver disorder, Lung affections, Mastitis, Measles, Milk-leg, Meningitis, Ovaries-affections of, Ozaena, Palpitation, Peritonitis, Perityphlitis, Phlebitis, Psoriasis palmaris, Purpura, Pyaemia, Remittent fever, Rheumatism, Scarlatina, Sleeplessness, Small-pox, Stings, Sunstroke, Syphilis, Tetanus, Thirst, Tongue-inflammation of; cancer of, Ulcer, Urticaria, Vaccination-effects of, Varicosis, Varicocele, Vomiting-bilious, White-leg, Whooping-cough, Yellow fever.

V. Symptoms-Particular (Nash-126)

1. Haemorrhage from every outlet of the body (Crotal. h., Acet. ac.). Even sweat is bloody.
2. Diphtheria-Chief remedy.
3. Nose bleed with great prostration.
4. Right sided remedy.

VI. Black Letter Symptoms (Tyler-335)

- Yellow colour of eyes.
- Blood oozes from ears.
- Bleeding from nose and all orifices of body.
- Tongue protruded.
- Black vomit.
- Jaundice: malignant jaundice; dark Haemorrhage from nose, mouth, etc. dark scanty urine.
- Easily tired by slightest exertion.
- Sudden and great prostration of vital force.
- Yellow Fever; haemorrhagic tendency, oozing of blood from every orifice and even pores of skin. Skin yellow, Vomiting of bile or blood.
- Foetid, bilious or bloody stools; liver tender, heart weak; faintness.
- Fever resulting from septic absorption and in purpuric cases of zymotic diseases; puerperal fever.
- Broken down Constitutions.

CROTON TIGLIUM

I. Introduction (Cow.-298)

Synonym: Tiglium offcinala.
Natural Order: Euphorbiaceae.
Common Name: Croton oil.
Habitat: Small tree in India and East.
Preparation: 1 part of pure croton oil dissolved in 99 parts of alcohol-2x.

1st provings were made by Dr. Hermann of Germany-(Pierce-430).

II. General Analysis (Cow.)

Acts especially upon mucous lining of intestinal tract and the skin: in the former, causing watery copious diarrhoea, and, in the latter, true eczema.

III. Suited to (Allen-113)

Copious watery diarrhoea (Verat.); acute eczema over whole body (Rhus t.); Intense itch but too tender to scratch, cough as soon as head touches pillow.

IV. Clinical (Clarke-I-618)

Cholera, Cholerine, Colds, Cornea-opacity of, Cough, Diarrhoea, Ear affections , Eczema, Eye affections, Hypopion, Keratitis, Neuralgia, Nipples painful, Ophthalmia, Proctalgia, Rheumatism, Rhus poisoning.

V. Symptoms-General (Nash-322)

1. Stool yellow, watery, coming out like a shot, all at once; < after least food or drink.
2. Excruciating pain, running from nipple to scapula; of same side when child nurses.

3. Eczema, esp. of the scrotum, itches intensely but is so sensitive to touch and sore that he can not scratch.

VI. **Symptoms-Particular** (Nash-322)

Most violent cathartic

1. Stool-Leads in following conditions of diarrhoea.
   (a) Yellow watery stool.
   Also found under (Apis., Coloc., China., Grat., Hyo., Nat. m.,
   Sul., Podo., Thuj.).
   (b) Sudden expulsion like a shot, all at once.
   Also under (Jatr., Grat., Podo., Thuj.).
   (c) Least food or drink—Arg. n., Ars.
   (d) Aloe.—rumbling before stool in the stomach.
   Crot. t.—Swashing in intestine as from water.
2. Pain in the same back side where child suckles nipple (Mastitis).
3. Eczema of Scrotum-sensitive to touch.

CUPRUM METALLICUM

I. Introduction (Cow.-300)

Common Name: Copper.
Preparation: Triturations of pure precipitated metallic copper.

It was first proved by Hahnemann (Chronic Diseases) (Pierce-431).

II. General Analysis (Cow.)

Acts prominently upon alimentary canal, producing Gastro-intestinal inflammation, colic, Diarrhoea, Vomiting, etc. Secondary action is upon nerve centres-Cramp, convulsion and paralysis. Chief characteristic-symptoms appear periodically and in groups.

III. Suited to (Allen-114)

Mental, physical, exhaustion from over exertion of mind and loss of sleep (Cocc., Nux. v.), attacks of unconquerable anxiety. Spasm and cramp appear in groups and periodically. Clonic spasms, Epilepsy.

IV. Clinical (Clarke-I-638)

After-pains, Angina pectoris, Asthma, Asthma Milleri, Cardialgia, Catarrh, Chlorosis, Cholera, Chorea, Convulsions, Cough, Cramps, Croup, Cyanosis, Dentition, Dyspnoea, Emissions, Epilepsy, Eruptions, Erysipelas, Fainting, Gastric disorders, Gout, Haematemesis, Herpes, Hysteria, Inflammations, Larynx-spasm of, Mania, Measles, Meningitis, Neuralgia, Palpitation, Paralysis, Pneumonia, Psoriasis, Ringworm, Sleeplessness, Spasms, Spinal irritation, Ulcer, Whooping-cough, Yellow fever.

V. **Symptoms-General** (Nash-265)

1. Spasm is the word characterising this remedy. Cramp or convulsion in Meningitis, Cholera, Cholera morbus, Whooping-cough. Scarlatina, etc.
2. Spasms begin in fingers and toes and, spreading from there, become general.
3. Mental or bodily exhaustion from over exertion of mind or loss of sleep.
4. Affections arising from suppressed skin troubles especially from acute exanthemata.

VI. **Symptoms-Particular** (Nash-265)

1. Spasm is the grand central characteristic, like collapse in Camph., evacuation and vomiting in Verat..
2. Spasm-(Zinc.) begins from finger to entire body.
3. Mental and bodily exhaustion from over exertion of mind or loss of sleep.
   Cocc.,
   Nux. v.
4. Whooping-cough-gets stiff, breathing ceases, Spasmodic twitchings, after a while consciousness returns slowly.

DIGITALIS PURPUREA

I. Introduction (Cow.-306)

Synonym: Digitalis Purpurea.
Natural Order: Scrophulariaceae.
Common Name: Foxglove.
Habitat: A beautiful plant common in Europe and the USA.
Preparation: Tincture from the fresh leaves of plant uncultivated and in second season.

Hahnemann first proved this remedy and said that its primary action was slowness of pulse and secondary a much quicker and smaller pulse (MMP Vol. 1425 symptoms) (Pierce-438).

II. General Analysis (Cow.)

Acts profoundly upon muscular substance of the heart and arteries, through pneumo-gastric and vaso-motor nerves causing debility, paralysis, arterial tension and intermittent pulse. In the heart it produces vigorous systolic contractions which become very irregular, causing one part of ventricle to dilate and other to contract. Finally the heart stops in systole. Its secondary action produces functional derangements of the brain, kidneys, and digestive organs. Chief characteristic extremely slow and intermittent pulse.

III. Suited to (Allen-117)

Pale face, death like appearance; blueness of skin, eyelids, lips tongue; sudden flushes of heat; intermittent pulse, occurring at climacteric motion. Sensation as if heart will stop, if she moved (Cocaine).

IV. Clinical (Clarke-I-664)

Amaurosis, Angina pectoris, Asthma, Bright's disease,

Cyanosis, Delirium tremens, Dropsy, Fever, Gonorrhoea, Headache, Heart affections, Hydrocele, Hydrocephalus, Impotence, Jaundice, Lung congested, Memory lost, Meningitis, Noises in head, Paraphimosis, Prostate enlarged, Ptyalism, Spermatorrhoea, Toothache, Urinary disorders, Vision disordered.

V. **Symptoms-General** (Nash-221)

1. Extremely slow, intermittent pulse, weak heart; or rapid, very irregular pulse.
2. Respiration; irregular, difficult, slow, deep or performed by frequent deep sighs; sometimes stops on dropping off to sleep.
3. Excessive jaundice, with slow, weak heart, and ashy white stools.
4. Faintness or sinking at the stomach, feels as if he would die if he moved.
5. Blueness of skin, eye lids; tongue; cyanosis, Distended veins on lids, ears, lips and tongue.

VI. **Symptoms-Particular** (Nash-221)

Heart remedy.

1. Very slow pulse, intermittent, pulse slow, may alternate with quick pulse. Spells of breathlessness, weakness, with purple face, bluish lips.
2. Heart would stop, sensation as if.
   If she moved-Dig.
   If she did not move-Gels.
   In any case it would cease-Lobel.
3. Breath fades way with sleep(223). Then wakes up with a gasp to catch it.
   Dig.,
   Grind.,
   Lach.
4. Blueness of skin, esp. eyelids, lips, tongue, nails, Cyanosis (323).
5. Respiration irregular, difficult, with frequent sighs (323).

6. Faintness or sinking at stomach—as if dying, great weakness and general sudden sinking of strength.
7. Jaundice—with ashy or perfectly colourless stools while urine as brown as lager beer, nausea, dropsy, vomiting (222), pulse slow, often dropped out a beat.

DIOSCOREA VILLOSA

I. Introduction (Cow.-309)

Synonym: Dioscorea.
Natural Order: Dioscoreaceae.
Common Name: Wild Yam.
Preparation: Tincture from the fresh roots.
Habitat: A perennial creeping plant of the USA.

It was named in honour of its discoverer, great Greek Botanist and Physician Dios Cariedes, and was first proved by Dr. Cushing of USA (Pierce-440).

II. General Analysis (Cow.)

It exerts its action mostly in the umbilical region through ganglionic nervous system, giving its most characteristic effects-severe pain simulating "bilious colic". It is different from its well known analogue Colocynthis in that while in Coloc. the patient bends double to get relief and feels that pressure would relief, in Diosc. most relief is obtained by stretching the body out.

III. Suited to (Allen-118)

Persons of feeble digestive powers, old or young, flatulence after meals, especially of tea drinkers, often subject to violent colic twisting as if grasped by a powerful hand. Griping pains about umbilicus. Colic pains < bending forward or lying > erect or bending backwards (Rev. of Coloc.).

IV. Clinical (Clarke-I-671)

Abdomen distended, Acne, Angina pectoris, Biliousness, Cholerine, Chorea, Colds, Colic, Constipation, Cough, Cramps, Diarrhoea, Dysentery, Dysmenorrhoea, Dyspepsia, Enteralgia, Flatulence, Gall-Bladder affections, Gastralgia, Haemorrhoids, Headache, Knee-pain in, Legs-pain in, Liver disorder, Lumbago, Mind-affections of, Neuralgia, Paronychia, Parotitis, Pregnancy-pyrosis of, Renal colic, Rheumatism, Sciatica, Side pain, Spinal irritation, Spleen-pain in, Smell disordered, Spermatorrhoea, Tea-effects of, Toothache, Whitlow.

V. **Symptoms-Particular** (Nash-470)

1. Colic at umbilicus radiates to all parts, even extremities.

DROSERA ROTUNDIFOLIA

I. Introduction (Cow.-313)

Synonym: Drosera Rotundifolia.
Natural Order: Droseraceæ.
Common Name: Round leaved sundew.
Habitat: A plant growing on turfy, mossy ground in Europe, America, North Asia.
Preparation: Tincture from the entire fresh plant.

It was first proved by Hahnemman (Pierce-443).

II. General Analysis (Cow.)

Acts powerfully upon respiratory system through influencing pneumogastric nerve, producing spasmodic cough which is characteristic of this drug, simulating that of Whooping-cough; can cause Tuberculosis in animals. Useful in respiratory affections, whooping cough with violent paroxysms, contraction of the throat and chest (315).

III. Suited to (Allen-121)

Whooping-cough with violent paroxysms, hardly able to breath < 6-7 AM. Deep sounding, hoarse barking cough (Verb.). Profuse Epistaxis during every paroxysm. "Minute gun" during day, Whooping at night (Coral. r.). Nocturnal cough of young people. Cough begins as head touches pillow (Bell., Hyo., Rum. c.), Cough < warmth, drinking, singing, Lying down, after midnight.

IV. Clinical (Clarke-I-679)

Amblyopia, Asthma, Bronchitis, Catarrh, Consumption, Cough, Coxalgia, Epilepsy, Haemorrhage, Headache, Laryngitis, Measles, Nausea, Phthisis, Sciatica, Vomiting, Whooping-cough.

V. Black Letter Symptoms
(Tyler 361-2)

- Crawling in larynx, which provokes coughing, with sensation as if a soft body was located there, with fine shooting therein to right side of gullet.
- Deep down in fauces (and on soft palate) a rough, scraping sensation with dryness exciting short cough, with yellow slimy expectoration and hoarseness of voice, so that it is only with an effort that he can speak in a deep base tone; at the same time he feels an oppression of the chest, as if something there kept back the air when he coughed and spoke. So the breath could not be expelled.
- Quivering in right shoulder, only when at rest.
- Paralytic pain in right hip joint and thigh, and in ankle joint. But in the latter rather as if dislocated, when walking, when he must limp on account of the pain.
- A single cutting stitch in the middle of the anterior aspect of left thigh recurring from time to time.
- A very acute pain, darts through the left side of the chest in fits.
- Great oppressive pain of the whole chest, especially on inspiration and expiration.
- Pain in small of back, as after long stooping.
- In the loin, above left hip, a digging, shooting pain.
- A drawing, tearing pain in both thighs.
- Lameness in small of back, as if from a cold.
- Eruption like nettle rash all over the body, without fever.
- Chill, commencing in, or spreading from back, not better for—warmth mostly towards evening.
- A fine cutting stitch in right calf, which comes when sitting and goes off on walking.
- Tearing pain in right ankle joint as if it were dislocated only when walking.
- Inflexibility of ankle joints—they are very stiff.
- A pain compounded of gnawing and shooting in the shafts of the bones of the arms, thighs and legs,

particularly severe in the joints, with severe stitches in the joints, less felt when moving than when at rest.

- Painful shooting pressure in the muscles of the upper and lower extremities at the same time, in every position.
- All the limbs are as if bruised and are also painful externally.
- Pain in all the limbs. He feels as if all were paralyzed.
- He is weak in the whole body, with sunken eyes and checks.
- Febrile rigor all over the body with heat in the face, but icy cold hands, without thirst.
- Restlessness—when reading he could not stick long to one subject, he must always go to something else.
- He is dejected about the malice of others on all hands, and at the same time disheartened and concerned about the future.
- Cough—the paroxysms follow each other so violently that he is scarcely able to get his breath.
- Rough, scraping, dry sensation deep on fauces, etc.

DULCAMARA

I. Introduction (Cow.-316)

Synonym: Solanum Dulcamara.
Natural Order: Solanaceae.
Common Name: Bitter Sweet, Woody Night Shade.
Habitat: A climbing shrubby plant growing in moist situations world over.
Preparation: Tincture from the fresh plant before flowering.

It was proved by Hahnemann (MMP 400 symptoms) (Pierce-444).

II. General Analysis (Cow.)

Acts especially upon mucous membranes and muscular tissues causing catarrhal and inflammatory rheumatic conditions like exposure to damp, rainy weather. Also acts upon lymphates and skin causing glandular enlargements and Eruption. Chief characteristic < Damp cold weather (Rhus t) (318).

III. Suited to (Allen-122)

Persons of phlegmatic, scrofulous constitutions, restless, irritable; patients living or working in a damp cold basement or milk dairy (Aran., Ars., Nat. s).Sudden changes in hot weather (Bry.). Exposure to cold, damp, rainy weather.

IV. Clinical (Clarke-686)

Adenitis, Angina faucium, Aphonia, Bladder affections, Blepharophathalmia, Catarrh, Cholera, Crusta lactea, Diarrhoea, Dropsy, Dysentery, Emaciation, Exostosis, Haemorrhage, Haemorrhoids, Hay-fever, Headache, Herpes, Influenza, Irritation, Lichen, Lumbago, Measles, Meningitis, Myalgia, Myelitis, Nettlerash, Neuralgia, Ophthalmia,

Paralysis, Pemphigus, Rheumatism, Scarlatina, Scrofula, Stammering, Stiff-neck, Thirst, Tibia-pains in, Tongue-affections of, Tonsilitis, Tumours, Typhoid, Urine-difficulty in passing; incontinence of, Warts, Whooping-cough.

V. **Symptoms-General** (Nash-360)

1. Affections caused by taking cold when the air changes suddenly from dry and warm to wet and cold.
2. Tongue and jaws become lame, if cold air or water chills them; neck stiff, back painful, loins lame, after taking cold.
3. Colic as if diarrhoea would occur, from taking cold.
4. Yellow watery diarrhoea with cutting colic before every stool, or dysentery from taking cold.
5. Most catarrhal states, with secretion of much mucous, caused by exposure to damp cold.
6. Dropsical swelling after suppressed sweat, or paralysis and other troubles from suppressed Eruption after taking cold.
7. Modalities; < from wet, cold weather after warm, dry, at nights and when at rest; > rising from a seat, motion; warmth in general, and dry weather.
8. Glands swell and hypertrophy on repeated exposures to cold, damp air, also acute and chronic tonsilitis.

VI. **Symptoms-Particular** (Nash-361)

1. Worse-from changes of weather from dry and warm to cold and (wet) damp.
   Dulc.-Sore throat with stiffness and lameness.
   Nat. s.-Asthma humidum, loose cough, rattling of mucous.
   Baryt. c.-resembles Dulc.
2. Effects of taking cold.
   Stiff neck (Baryt. c.), painful back (Rhus t.) and limbs.
3. Sore throat and quinsy-Tongue paralyzed.
   Dulc., Baryt. c.
4. Asthma Humidum (Loose cough).
   Dulc.,
   Dulc. (Reverse of Acon.).

5. Diarrhoea and colic-in hot weather, when days or nights become suddenly cold-Dysentery.

VII. Black Letter Symptoms
(Tyler-365-66)

- Scald head, thick brown crusts with reddish borders, on forehead, temples and chin; bleeding when scratched.
- Humid eruption on cheeks.
- Thick, brown yellow crusts on face, Crusta lactea.
- Thick crusts all over body.
- Warts and eruption on face.
- Warts on hands and backs of fingers.
- Warts, fleshy or large, smooth, on dorsa of hands and on face.
- Tongue paralysed from cold, yet talk incessantly.
- Inarticulate speech from swollen tongue.
- Colic: as from taking cold: as if diarrhoea would occur.
- Colic such as is usually caused by wet cold weather.
- Yellow watery diarrhoea with tearing,cutting colic before very evacuation.
- Mucous diarrhoea, alternately yellow and greenish.
- Diarrhoea from cold, or changing from warm to cold, especially cold damp weather.
- Catarrhal troubles caused by cold damp weather.
- Cough from damp cold atmosphere, or from getting wet. Must cough a long time to expel phlegm.
- Ill smelling perspiration.
- Ear ache, nausea, buzzing worse at night.
- Earache the whole night preventing sleep.
- Great opprenive pain of the whole chest, esp on inspiration and expiration.
- Pain in swell of back, as after long stooping.
- In the loin, above left hip, a digging shooting pain.
- A drawnig tearing pain in both thighs.
- Lamenen in swell of back, as if from a cold.
- Eruptrons like nettle rash all over body, without fear.
- Chill commencing in, or spreading from back, not better for warmath, mostly towards evening.

EQUISETUM HYEMALE

I. Introduction (Cow.-320)

Synonym: Equisetum Hyemale.
Natural Order: Equisetaceae.
Common Name: Scouring Bush.
Habitat: An indigenous leafless plant.
Preparation: Tincture from the fresh whole plant.

It was first proved by Dr. Smith in 1876 (Pierce-447).

II. General Analysis (Cow.)

Acts exclusively upon urinary organs giving rise to dysuria and symptoms, indicating a specific influence over the mucous lining of the bladder, with great vasical irritation pain and tenderness, pain not > by micturation, < just after. Nocturnal enuresis of children. Weakness of bladder, incontinence of urine, dribbling esp. in old men and insane. Haematuria, Gonorrhoea , Gleet (321).

III. Suited to (Allen-124)

Severe dull pain in bladder not better after urinating. Frequent and intolerable urging to urinate with severe pain at the close of urination (Berb. v., Sarsa., Thuj.). Sharp, cutting pain in urethra while urinating.

IV. Clinical (Clarke-I-707)

Cystitis, Dropsy, Enuresis, General paralysis, Gleet, Gonorrhoea, Gravel, Haematuria, Urine-retention of.

V. Symptoms-Particular (Nash-422)

Urinary problems.

1. Usually indicated after Canth., in Enuresis, Mucous in excess (Chim.).

Canth.-Scanty urine with burning.

Equis.-Profuse urine with burning, with excess of mucous (Chima).

2. Severe pain at close of urination sometimes.

Berb. v.,
Nat. m.,
Sarsa.,
Thuj.

EUPATORIUM PERFOLIATUM

I. Introduction (Cow.-324)

Synonym: Eupatorium Cormatum.
Natural Order: Compositeae.
Common Names: Thoroughwort, Bone set Agne weed.
Habitat: A hairy perennial plant throughout Canada and the USA.
Preparation: Tincture of the entire fresh plant just in bloom.

It was first proved by Drs. Williamson and Naid Hard in 1846 (Pierce-450).

II. General Analysis (Cow.)

Acts upon gastro-hepatic system, fibrous tissues and bronchial mucous membranes. Its name break bone is derived from its characteristic symptoms—great aching and soreness in the bones, soreness (deep) in muscles. Bilious derangement of a malarial character.

III. Suited to (Allen-125)

The diseases of old people, worn out constitutions, esp. from inebriety, Cachexia (constitutional disorder) from prolonged or frequent attack of bilious/intermittent Fever. Bone pains (Bry., Merc. c.) more severe and general better adapted. Painful soreness of eyeballs.

IV. Clinical (Clarke-I-127)

Anus-herpes of, Back pains, Bilious fever, Bones-pain in, Cough, Dengue, Diarrhoea, Fracture, Gout, Hiccough, Hoarseness, Indigestion, Influenza, Intermittent fever, Jaundice, Liver-soreness of, Measles, Mouth-cracks of, Ophthalmia, Relapsing fever, Remittent fever, Rheumatism, Ringworm, Spotted fever, Syphilitic pains, Thirst, Wounds.

V. Symptoms-General (Nash-414)

1. Painful soreness of eye balls; Coryza, aching in every bone, prostration in epidemic of influenza (La Grippe.).
2. Deep hard achings, as if in the bones, with sore bruised feeling all over, back, arms, wrists and legs.
3. Vomiting of bile between chill and heat, chill 7 to 9 AM.
4. Hoarseness in the morning, with soreness in the chest when coughing; holds it with hands.

VI. Symptoms-Particular (Nash-415-16)

1. Bruised feeling, as if broken, all over body (Arn., Bellis., Pyr.), with deep hard aching as if in bones.
2. With soreness of flesh and bones, painful soreness, in wrists, arms, forearms, as if broken. Limbs-stiff and sore when rising to walk.

   Eup. perf. is popularly known as 'Bone-set'.
3. Leading indicators are
   (a) Chill -7-9 AM.
   (b) Intense aching in the bones before chill.
   (c) Vomiting of bile between chill and heat.
4. Hoarseness in the morning.

   Caust.—more burning, rawness.

   Eup. perf.—more soreness in the chest.

   Ran. b.—pain in chest when walking.
5. Supports chest when coughing, to avoid hurt.

   Eup. perf., Bry., Dros., Kreas., Nat. s., Sep. (Sul.-when these medicines fail.)

   Bry. is the near analogue of Eup. perf.

EUPHRASIA

I. Introduction (Cow.-331)

Synonym: Euphrasia officinalis.
Natural Order: Scrophulariaceae.
Common Name: Eye bright.
Habitat: A small annual plant growing in meadows and on borders of the forests in Europe.
Preparation: Tincture from the fresh plant, omitting roots. It was proved by Hahnemann (Pierce-452).

II. General Analysis (Cow.)

Acts almost entirely upon mucous membrane especially of eyelids and upper portion of the respiratory tract. Chief characteristic—Flu-like catarrhal infection with watery secretion.

III. Suited to (Allen-126)

Catarrhal affections of eye and nose. Profuse acrid lachrymation. Profuse bland nasal catarrh (Both reverse of All. c.). Eye waters all the time. Bad effects of fall injury (Arn.). Cough < day > night (Nash).

IV. Clinical (Clarke-I-741)

Blepharitis, Cataract, Colds, Condylomata, Conjunctivitis, Cough, Eye affections, Glandular swellings, Granular lids, Influenza, Iritis, Lachrymation, Lips-stiffness of, Measles, Nasal catarrh, Nose-cancer of, Parotitis, Phlyctenulae, Pimples, Ptosis, Prolapsus ani, Prostate-affections of, Scrofula, Staphyloma, Sycosis.

V. Symptoms-Particular (Nash-444)

1. Eye-centre of action.

2. Severe fluent Coryza in cold with cough.
   Ars.,
   All. c.-Nasal discharge acrid, lachrymation bland.
   Merc. c.,
   Euph.-Nasal discharge bland, lachrymation acrid.
3. Measles with watery Eyes and fluent Coryza.
   Euph.-Best suited.
4. Sticky Mucous on cornea(Eye) removed by winking (eyelids are involved).
   Euph.,
   Ars.,
   Apis.,
   Rhus t.
5. Cough sometimes dry but generally loose. < during day, not troublesome at night.

FERRUM METALLICUM

I. Introduction (Cow.-333)

Synonym: Ferum Metallicum.
Preparation: Triturations of pure Iron reduced by Hydrogen.

It was first proved by Hahnemann who recorded 295 symptoms in MMP. (Pierce-454).

II. General Analysis (Cow.)

Ferr. acts predominantly upon the blood so as to produce a debilitating and disorganizing effect. It produces a condition like anaemia, in the treatment of which it is the most important medicine. Its primary effect is to increase RBCs, but continued use results in the opposite.

III. Suited to (Allen-127)

Persons of sanguine temperament, petty, quarrel some, least contradiction angers (Anac., Cocc., Ign.) > mental exertion. Irritable-slight noises like crackling of paper drive him to despair(Asar., Tarent. cub.) Women who are week, delicate, chlorotic, yet have a fiery red face. Extreme paleness of face, lips, and mucous membrane which become red and flushed on least pain, emotion or exertion.

IV. Clinical (Clarke-I-753)

Anaemia, Aphonia, Asthma, Biliousness, Catalepsy, Chlorosis, Chorea, Consumption (Ferr., Acet. ac.), Cough, Cramps, Debility, Diarrhoea, Enuresis diurna, Fever-intermittent, Goitre-exophthalmic, Gonorrhoea, Haemorrhage, Heart-affections of; palpitation of, Hectic, Hydrocephalus, Kidney-affections of, Lienteria, Menstruation disordered, Neuralgia, Paralysis of viscera, Pregnancy-affections of, Rectum-prolapse of, Rheumatism, Shoulder-affections of,

Spasms, Syphilis, Toothache, Urine-incontinence of, Vertigo.

V. Symptoms-General (Nash-299)

1. Anaemia with great paleness of all the mucous membranes; with sudden fiery red flushing of the face.
2. Profuse haemorrhage from any organ; haemorrhagic diathesis; blood light with dark clots; coagulates easily.
3. Local congestions and inflammations, with hammering, pulsating pains; veins full, flushed face, alternates with paleness.
4. Canine hunger, alternates with complete lose of appetite.
5. Regurgitations or Eructation or vomiting of food at night that has stayed in the stomach all day; undigested painless diarrhoea.
6. Red face during chill.
7. Modalities: < after eating and drinking; while at rest, especially sitting still; > walking slowly around.

VI. Symptoms-Particular (Nash-299-304)

1. Red Face-on least emotion or exertion, rush of blood to head.
2. Hammering, beating, pulsating pains in head.
   Bell.,
   China,
   Nat. m.,
   Glon.
3. Great paleness of mucous membranes especially of cavity of mouth.
4. > Walking, in spite of weakness which obliges patient to lie down.
5. Menses too soon, too profuse, too long lasting. Menstrual flow watery, pale weakening, ringing in the ears (China.), debilitating.
6. Haemorrhage, in anaemia with above peculiar symptoms.

7. Canine hunger alternates with complete loss of appetite (China.).

   Nat. m.-meat agrees (Opposite of Ferr.).

   Ferr.-meat does not agree. Beer or Tea disagrees. Food lies in the stomach all day is vomited at night. Wants bread and butter.

8. Undigested painless stool at night or after eating or drinking.

   Crot. t,

   China.,

   Ferr.-Bowels feel sore, as if bruised. China-more flatulence than Ferr.

9. Slow walking about relieves (Puls.)-in all diseases.
10. Flushed and Red face during chill-one of few medicines where it is found.
11. Cough with vomiting of food-one of the best remedies.
12. Regurgitation of food or eructation after eating.

VII. Black Letter Symptoms

(Tyler-370-1)

- Vertigo on rising suddenly; things grew black; had to lean against something; or fall; with nausea. Prostration lethargy; as if balancing to and fro; as when on water; when walking over water, like when crossing a bridge; when descending, with disposition to fall forward.
- Headache for 2 or 4 days every two or three weeks; hammering, beating, pulsating pains. Must lie down in bed; with aversion to eating and drinking.
- "Morbus Basedowii" especially after suppression of menses; protruding eyes; enlarged thyroid; palpitation; excessive nervousness.
- Epistaxis in anaemic children, with frequent changing colour of face.
- Extreme paleness of Face, which becomes red and flushes on least emotion, pain or exertion.
- Face flushes easily on least excitement or exertion.
- Canine Hunger alternating with loss of appetite.

- Anorexia; extreme dislike to all food.
- Vomiting only of food, immediately after eating.
- After eating eructation and regurgitations of food, without nausea or inclination to vomit.
- Vomiting of food immediately after midnight, followed by aversion of food and dread of open air.
- Cramp-like pain in stomach.
- Frequent Diarrhoea; stools watery, with or without tenesmus and preceded or not by pain, but always with much flatulence and more frequent after taking food or drink.
- Undigested stools at night, or while eating or drinking.
- The thread worms seem to be increased by it.
- Involuntary Urination at night, also when walking about by day.
- Nocturnal seminal emissions.
- Menses too soon, too profuse, too long lasting, with fiery red face, ringing in ears; flow pale, watery, debilitating.
- Vomiting of pregnancy; suddenly leaves table and with one effort vomits all the food taken, appetite not impaired thereby; can sit down and eat again.
- Difficult Breathing, oppression of Chest, as if some one pressed with hand upon it.
- Contractive spasm in chest and cough, only when moving and walking.
- Spasmodic cough after meals with vomiting of all food taken.
- Whooping-cough, child vomits food with every coughing spell; great pallor and weakness.
- Scanty, thin, frothy expectoration with streaks of blood.
- Haemoptysis; of onanists and consumptives; from severe exertion; from suppressed menses.
- Erethitic chlorosis, worse in winter.
- Anaemia masked behind plethora and congestions; pale colour of mucous membranes, with a nun's murmur.
- "Nun's murmur" in veins.

- Restless; must walk slowly about.
- The pain forces him to get up out of bed at night and walk slowly about.
- Emaciation.
- Red parts become white.
- Anaemia, from whatever cause, chlorisis of defective menstruation or simple poverty of blood induced by Haemorrhage, deficiency of air, light and suitable food, or of exhausting diseases.
- Cholorosis after great loss of blood.
- General haemorrhagic diathesis, Haemorrhophilia.
- Sleeps uneasily; is long awake before falling asleep again.

FERRUM PHOSPHORICUM

I. Introduction (Cow.-340)

Synonym: Phosphate of Iron.

Preparation: Trituration. It is comparatively a recent medicine. Proved by Dr. JC Morgan in 1876 (Pierce-460).

II. General Analysis (Cow.)

It represents many points, combined both of Iron and Phosphorus, and is a fever and inflammation remedy which occupies middle place between Acon. and Gels. It is recommended in the first stage of all inflammations before exudation has set in (IInd stage-Kali chlor.); sweat, thirst and heat which does not relieve the pain, useful for results of taking cold esp. from suppressed perspiration.

III. Clinical (Clarke-I-770)

Anus-prolapse of, Bladder-paralysis of, Bronchitis, Colic, Cough, Croup, Cystitis, Debility, Delirium tremens, Diabetes, Diarrhoea, Dyspepsia, Dysentery, Ear affections, Erysipelas, Fever, Frost-bite, Gastritis, Gonorrhoea, Haematemesis, Haemoptysis, Haemorrhage, Hands swollen, Heart-palpitation of, Inflammation, Injuries, Intermittent fever, Kidney-Bright's disease of, Measles, Mumps, Naevus, Neuralgia, Nose-bleed, Phthisis haemorrhagica, Pleurisy, Pneumonia, Raynaud's disease, Rheumatism, Sprain, Styes, Tarsal cysts, Urine-incontinence of, Veins-varicose , Vomiting, Whooping-cough.

IV. Nash—Particulars

1. First Stage of inflammation (Acon, Bell.) (32), Tousillitis (142).
2. Quinice Cachoxia (51).
3. Haemorrhags from all out lets (crot, Sul. A) (47), of bright blood (259).
4. First stage of dysentery with blood (259).
5. Night sweats of weak and anaemic (259).

FLUORIC ACID

I. Introduction (Cow.-341)

Synonym: Hydrofluoric Acid.
Preparation: One part of pure Fluoric Acid dissolved in 99 parts of alcohol in gutta percha vials giving 2x.
It was first proved under Dr. Hoering's directions (Pierce-462).

II. General Analysis (Cow.)

Acts upon vegetative system (a tissue remedy), mucous surfaces, glandular structure, bones, and broken down conditions. Chief characteristics (i) Ulcer/ tumours better by cold application. (ii) > as if she can walk for ever. (iii) Fistula lachrymalis, Fistula dentalis and fistula of the jaw bones. Teeth sensitive to touch (Pierce-463).

III. Suited to (Allen-128)

Complaints of old age, or of premature old age; in syphilitic mercurial dyscrasia, young people look old.

IV. Clinical (Clarke-I-782)

Abscess, Alcoholism, Alopecia, Apoplexy, Bone affections, Brain-atrophy of, Cicatrix, Coccygodynia, Decubitus, Dropsy, Eye affections, Fistula, Gleet, Goitre, Gonorrhoea, Haemorrhoids, Hair falling off, Hands perspiring, Headache, Hydrocele, Liver indurated, Locomotor ataxy, Naevus, Nose-inflammation of, Nymphomania, Otorrhoea, Peritonitis, Perspiration, Pityriasis, Satyriasis, Splenalgia, Suppuration, Syphilis, Teeth defective, Toothache, Tongue ulcerated, Varicosis, Veins diseased, Whitlow.

GELSEMIUM

I. Introduction (Cow.-346)

Synonym: Gelsemium Semper virens.
Natural Order: Loganiacae.
Common Name: Yellow Jessamine.
Habitat: A climbing plant indigenous to Southern United States.
Preparation: Tincture from the fresh root.

It was first proved by Dr. JM Henry in 1852, and by Dr. EM Hab in 1862 (Pierce-466).

II. General Analysis (Cow.)

Produces prostration, spinal convulsion, and paralysis, lowering the force and rate of heart finally paralysing respiration, Consciousness is always preserved. Leading expressions-low nervous condition with drowsiness, languor, quite and erethism.

III. Suited to (Allen-129)

Children, young people, especially women of hysterical temperament (Croc., Ign.). Complete relaxation and prostration of whole muscular system with entire motor paralysis. Bad effects from fright, fear sudden emotions (Ign.) (from pleasant surprises-Coff.). Utter lack of courage.

IV. Clinical (Clarke-I-805)

Amaurosis, Anterior crural neuralgia, Aphonia, Astigmatism, Bilious fever, Brain-affections of, Cerebro-spinal meningitis, Choroiditis, Colds, Constipation, Convulsions, Deafness, Dengue fever, Diarrhoea, Diphtheria, Dupuytren's contraction, Dysentery, Dysmenia, Emotions-effects of, Epilepsy, Eye affections, Fever, Fright, Gonorrhoea , Hay-fever, Headache, Heat-effects of, Heart disease, Hydrosalpingitis, Hysteria, Influenza, Intermittent fever, Jaundice, Labour, Liver-affections of, Locomotor ataxy, Mania, Measles, Meningitis, Menstruation-painful; suppressed, Metrorrhagia, Myalgia, Neuralgia, Nystagmus, Oesophagus-constriction of, Paralysis, Paralysis agitans, Paraplegia, Pregnancy-albuminuria of, Ptosis, Puerperal convulsions, Remittent fever, Retina-detachment of, Rheumatism, Sexual excess-effects of, Sleep disordered, Spasms, Sun-headaches, Sunstroke, Teething, Tic douloureux, Tobacco-effect of, Tongue-affections of, Toothache, Tremors, Uterine affections, Vertigo, Voice lost, Writer's cramp.

V. **Symptoms-General** (Nash-252)

1. Complete relaxation and prostration of the whole muscular system, with almost or entire motor paralysis.
   Eyelids droop; muscles refuse to obey the will.
2. Trembling of hands or lower extremities if he attempts to move; must lie still.
3. Mental faculties dull, can't think; with dull red face.
4. Susceptibility to mental disturbance, excitement or emotion; causes diarrhoea.
5. Dull, tired, prostrating headache at base of brain; wants head high, sometimes > by profuse urination.
6. Vertigo with blurred vision; dilated pupils; double sight; sense of intoxication.
7. Nervous chill, violent shaking with no sense of coldness.
8. Desire to be quiet; feels too weak to move. Children; fear of falling, seize the nurse, grab the crib, especially in intermittents.
9. Slow, weak pulse of old age.
10. Great heaviness of the eyelids; cannot keep them open.
11. Fears that unless constantly on the move, the heart will cease beating.
12. General deep-seated muscular pain with prostration (la grippe).

VI. Symptoms-Particular (Nash-253-257)

1. Pre-eminently a nerve remedy (254).
   Trembling remedy
2. Trembling external with weakness, drowsy (Pic. ac., Gels.), hands, legs tremble. Wants to lie down so weak (Pic. ac.).
3. Eyelids droop, later it may develop into paralysis so weak. Can't guide his fingers and feet while sensorium remain clear. He knows what he wants to do but can't. Muscles don't obey the will.

   Sep., Caust., Gels. } Eye lids droop.
4. Diarrhoea due to sudden excitement or emotion.-Gels.
5. Dizziness-blurred vision, intoxicated, pupils dilated.-Gels.
6. Downward motion scares-Bor., Gels.
7. Flow of urine-Lac def.-profuse urine during headache. No vomiting or nausea, as in Iris v., Sang., Lac def.
8. Fever Dull, remittent, child does not want to move because of weakness. It stands between Acon. and Verat., also Bap. and Bell.

   Bap.-Like Gels. prostration but typhoid tongue etc. not so strong. Patient falls asleep when trying to answer question, offensive sweat stool and urine of Bap. are not in Gels.

   Bell.-Like Gels. congestion of brain, pupils dilated, but not as intense as in Bell.
9. Nervous chill-one of the best remedies.

   Gels.-Chill runs up and down the back in wave like succession.

   Great shaking and chattering of teeth, with no objective coldness.

   Wants to be held because he shakes so.
10. Torpid, sleepy, dreads movement. Mental faculties are dull-can't fix attention or think clearly.

11. Susceptibility to mental disturbance, such as sudden excitement or emotion, bad news or fright-it causes diarrhoea.
12. Headache-dull, tired headache, wants to lie down with head high and perfectly still, < mental labour, tobacco, lying with head low and in heat of sun (Glon., Lach., Lyss., Nat. c.) Sometimes relieved by profuse urination. Headache from passive congestion-then pain begins in the occiput and spreads all over the head. Lac def. has also profuse flow of urination, pain is not so markedly relieved.

VII. Black Letter Symptoms (Tyler-385)

- Dullness of mind, alleviated on profuse emission of watery urine.
- Incapacity to think, or fix the attention.
- Dizziness of head and blurred vision gradually increased, so that all objects appeared very indistinct.
- Head felt very light.
- Heaviness of head alleviated on profuse emission of watery urine.
- Sensitive bruised sensation of brain.
- Drooping of the eyelids.
- Difficulty in opening the eyelids, or in keeping them upon.
- Dimness of sight and vertigo.
- Smoky appearance before the eyes, with pain above them.
- Objects appeared double.
- Heavy besotted face, flushed and hot to touch.
- No control over lower jaw, it wagged sideways.
- Numbness of tongue. Tongue so thick, he could hardly speak.
- Tired to swallow, but he could not.
- Frequent emission of clear, limpid urine, with seeming relief to dullness and heaviness of head.
- Severe, sharp labour like pains in uterine region, extending to back and hips.
- Irregular beating of heart, palpitation of heart. Pulse markedly affected.

- Trembling in all the limbs.
- Lost control of limbs, could not direct their movements with precision.
- Fatigue of the lower limbs, after slight exercise.
- Trembling and weakness (accompanying profuse urination).
- Complete relaxation of whole muscular system with entire motor paralysis.
- Listless and languid.
- Easily fatigued, especially the lower limbs.
- Weakness and trembling through the whole system.
- Chilliness, especially along the spine.

GLONOINE

I. Introduction (Cow.-352)

Common Name: Nitro Glycerine.
Preparation: Tincture made by dissolving 1 part of this medicine in 9 parts of alcohol IX dilution subsequent with Alcohol. This medicine, a mixture of glycerine on nitric and sulphuric acids was discovered by Dr. Sobraro in Paris.

It was first proved by Dr. Herning in 1848-49 (Pierce-473-474).

II. General Analysis (Cow.)

Acts upon medulla oblongata and pneumo-gastric, producing active (Amyl Nitrite-passive) cerebral hyperaemia (excess of blood), and palpitation of heart, former resembling symptoms of exposures to sun's rays to intense sunstroke, without fever and inflammation which are ever with cerebral disorders of Acon., Bell. Chief expression is throbbing fullness in the brain (Not pain).

III. Suited to (Allen-131)

Nervous temperament, plethoric, florid, (flushed) sensitive women. Bad effects of mental excitement. Head trouble when heat falls on head (gaslight, heat of sun) etc.

IV. Clinical (Clarke-I-824)

Angina pectoris, Aphasia, Apoplexy, Brain-congestion of, Bright's disease, Convulsions, Epilepsy, Epistaxis, Fear-effects of, Goitre, Headache, Heart-affections of; palpitation of; Jarring-effects of, Location-sense of lost, Mania, Meningitis, Menses suppressed, Neuralgia, Paralysis, Rheumatism, Sciatica, Sea-sickness, Snow-headache, Sun-headaches, Sunstroke, Toothache, Trauma.

V. Symptoms-General (Nash-450)

1. Sudden local congestion, especially to head and chest; bursting headache rising up from neck, with great throbbing and sense of expansion as if to burst; cannot bear the least jar.
2. Can't bear anything on the head, especially hat; or pressure as of a hat.
3. Over-heating in the sun, or sunstroke.

VI. Symptoms-Particular (Nash-450-3)

1. Headache-Throbbing visible in carotid, sensation of waves in brain; with the pulse.
   Bell. = Glon.
   (i) Fullness, pain and throbbing-Bell.
   Gel-more intense onset, but subsides rapidly.
   (ii) Congestion-Gels.-Ist or congestive stage.
   Bell.-even after the congestive stage.
   (iii) Better bending head backward-Bell.
   Worse bending head backward-Gels.
   (iv) < Hair cut-Bell.
   < Head in covered-Gel.
   (v) < Lying down-Bell.
   Gels.-sometimes worse, sometimes > lying still.
   (vi) < Jar-least Jar-Gels. Carries head very carefully.
   (vii) More disturbance in head-Bell.
   in chest-Gels.
2. Great congestion to head (From delayed Menses)
   Meli.-Great congestion with pain and fullness.
   "Glowing redness of face".
   Profuse Epistaxis. > head symptoms.
3. Loses ways in well known streets.
4. Convulsion with Albumin in urine.
5. Sunstroke-Bad effects of radiate heat such as open Coal fire. (453).
6. Warm Room increases headache, warm bed face ache.
7. Burning between shoulders-Lyc., Phos., Gels.
   (opp: Amm. mur., Lach., Anthrac.).

VII. Black Letter Symptoms
(Tyler-388-9)

- Well-known streets seem strange; way home too long.
- Disinclined to speak; would hardly answer.
- A distinct feeling of pulse in Head. Throbbing in front of head.
- Immediately a sensation as if head were too large.
- Head felt enormously large.
- Pressure and throbbing in temples.
- Pressure and pain from within out in both temples.
- Fullness in head, and throbbing without pain.
- Head very full; Pulse full and quick.
- As if he were hanging with head downward, and as if there were a great rush of blood into head in consequence.
- As if blood were mounting to head.
- As if skull were too small; and brain attempting to burst it.
- Afraid to shake his head lest it drop to pieces.
- Holds head with both hands; presses sinciput.
- Shocks in brain, synchronous with every pulsation of arteries.
- Undulating sensation in head.
- Throbbing in head; in temples; in temporal arteries which were raised and felt like whipcords.
- Sensation of fullness, vertex and forehead.
- Shaking the head increases the headache.
- Headache on damp, rainy days; after taking cold; after much sitting, and mental exertion.
- Red injected hot Eyes during headache, with wild expression.
- Throbbing pain in all the teeth.
- Throbbing in whole body.
- Intense congestion of brain induced in plethoric constitutions by sudden Suppression of Menses or appearing instead of menses.
- Headaches occurring after profuse uterine haemorrhage.

- Rush of blood to head in pregnant women, with pale face and loss of consciousness.
- Violent palpitation of Heart, with throbbing carotids, pulsating headache in forehead and between temples.
- Blood seems to rush to heart and mount rapidly into head.
- Epileptic Convulsion, with congestion to head and heart.
- Bad effects from being exposed immediately to sun's rays.
- (In fever) flushes of heat; waves of heat upwards.

GRAPHITES

I. Introduction (Cow.-356)

Synonym: Plumbago, Carbo Mineralis.
Common Name: Black Lead.
Preparation: Triturations.

It was first proved by Hahnemann-1140 symptoms in Chronic Diseases (Pierce-477).

II. General Analysis (Cow.)

Acts especially upon skin, lymphatics, digestive system, and sexual organs. Upon skin it produces a moist, scaly eruption Dry and scaly (Lyc.) hard scabs-(Mez.). Scabs easily torn but bleed (Hep. s.). Also acts upon sexual system esp. upon ovaries and testes.

III. Suited to (Allen-133)

Women, inclined to obesity, who suffer from habitual constipation with a history of delayed menstruation. "What Puls. is at puberty, Graph. is at climacteric".

IV. Clinical (Clarke-I-835)

Acne, Amenorrhoea, Anus-affections of, Blepharitis, Breasts-indurated; cancer of, Cancer, Catarrh, Chaps, Chlorosis, Colic, Constipation, Deafness, Dropsy, Dysmenorrhoea, Ears-affections of, Eczema, Epistaxis, Erysipelas, Eye affections, Face-erethema of, Feet-affections of, Fissures, Gastralgia, Glandular swellings, Gleet, Gravel, Haemorrhoids, Headache, Herpes, Hydrocele, Influenza, Irritation, Lachrymal duct inflamed, Leucorrhoea, Lips cracked, Liver indurated, Menstruation disordered, Mentagra, Nails diseased, Noises in head, Nose affections, Nose-bleed, Obesity, Ovarian tumours, Paralysis, Parotitis, Pityriasis, Priapism, Pruritus vaginae, Psoriasis, Ptosis, Rectum-affections of,

Rhus poisoning, Scar inflamed, Scrofula, Seminal emissions, Skin-affections of, Smell disordered, Stomach-cramp in, Sycotic diathesis, Syphilis, Trichiasis, Tumours, Ulcer, Urinary disorders, Uterus-cancer of, Vaccination-effects of, Wens, Whooping-cough, Worms, Zona.

V. **Symptoms-General** (Nash-283)

1. Eruption on the skin, oozing out a thick, honey like fluid.
2. Mucous outlets; eyelids inflamed, with pustules; ears discharge, moist sore places behind ears; mouth cracked in corners; anus, eruption, itching, fissured.
3. Nails grow thick, cracked, out of shape.
4. Constipation; stools knotty, large lumps, united by mucous threads. One of the best remedies for fissure ani, pain after stool, soreness after wiping it (286). Often eczema around anus.
5. Diarrhoea; stools brown fluid, mixed with undigested substances, and of an intolerably foetid odour.
6. Sad and despondent; inclined to weep, thinks of nothing but death.
7. Especially adapted to persons inclined to obesity; particularly females who delay menstruation.
8. Hears better when in a noise; when riding in a carriage or car: when there is a rumbling sound.
9. Sensation of cobweb on forehead; tries hard to brush it off.

VI. **Symptoms-Particular** (Nash-284-287)

A powerful anti Psoric (Lyc., Psor., Caust., etc.).

1. Skin-Eruption-oozing a thick honey like fluid, on any part of body, but esp. on or behind ears, head, face, genitals, eyelids.

   Graph.,
   Sul.,
   Psor.,
   Caust.

2. Brown fluid stool, mixed with undigested substance and of intolerable foetid odour.

   Psor. } stools are similar, but nature of eruption,
   Graph. } which is different in these two, will decide.

   China (Brown, loose, foetid stools)-if no eruption, but extreme weakness from long continued drain or loss of fluid.

3. Eczema of Eyelids.

   Graph.,–enptions most, lids fissured, scaly crusty.

   Staph.,–second to graph.

   Sul. (Lid margin very red) Graph. leads in eyelid eczema.

4. Nails thick grow out of shape (both finger and toe nails).

   Graph.-Cracks or Fissure in the ends of fingers (Nipples, labial commissures of anus).

   Sarsa.,

   Petr.-Fissure between toes (Graph.).

5. Herpetic Dyscrasia-one of best for Wens in persons.
6. In menses Graph. resembles Puls.
7. Menses are scanty and delayed in Graph. but profuse and soon in Calc. c.
8. Sensation of Cobweb on forehead.

   Pointers (1) Peculiar tendency to obesity.
   (2) Catarrhic glutinous eruption.

9. Generally tends to constipation than diarrhoea. Stools-knotty and large sometimes united by mucous threads and mucous often follows stool.
10. Eczema around anus.
11. Lumps in the breast, of suspicious appearance, go away under action of this remedy.

VII. Black Letter Symptoms (Tyler-398-400)

- Sadness, with thought of nothing but death.
- Despondent. Feels miserable, unhappy.
- Apprehensiveness, with inclination to weep. Music makes her weep.
- Pain as if Head were numb and pithy.

- Pain as if constricted, esp. occiput.
- Falling of hair of scalp. Itching on scalp.
- Much scaliness of head, which causes distressing itching and becomes a scurf, which disappears on washing and then is humid.
- Eruption on vertex, painful to touch and humid.
- Eczema capitis of entire scalp, forming massive dirty crusts which met the hair. Painful and sore to touch.
- Falling out of hair of scalp.
- Eyes: very inflamed margins of lids.
- Inflammation of the external canthi, sore and fissured; bleed easily. Edges of lids much inflamed. Dry mucous on lashes.
- Deafness-hears better in a noise or riding in a carriage.
- Moist and sore places behind both Ears.
- Soreness in Nose on blowing it.
- Nose painful internally. Dryness of nose. Nose stopped with badly smelling mucous.
- Dry scabs in nose, with sore, cracked and ulcerated nostrils.
- Smell abnormally acute: can't tolerate flowers.
- Constant sensation of cobweb on Face.
- Soreness and cracking of lips and nostrils, as from cold.
- Burning blisters lower side and tip of tongue.
- Taste of rotten eggs which nauseates.
- Constrictive pains in Stomach; better eating.
- Aversion to animal food; to fish: to cooked food.
- Sweet things are disgusting and nauseous.
- Burning pains radiate through Abdomen. Heaviness in abdomen.
- Great distension of abdomen.
- Full abdomen as from accumulation and incarceration of flatus.
- Pain in upper abdomen.
- Hardness in region of liver.
- Smarting sore pain in Anus on wiping it.
- Itching in anus.
- Stools brown, fluid, with undigested substances; of

intolerable odour.

- Stool dark coloured, half digested, of an intolerable odour.
- Stool lumpy, conjoined with threads of mucous.
- Sticking in anus (with hard stool and much urging).
- Discharge of mucus from rectum.
- Haemorrhoids with burning rhagades at anus.
- Urine becomes turbid and deposits white sediment.
- Profuse leucorrhoea of very white mucus; acrid; excoriating.
- Itching of pudenda before menstruation.
- Menstruation delayed.
- Hard cicatrices remaining after mammary abscess, retarding flow of milk.
- Cancer of mammae, from old cicatrices, which had remained after repeated abscesses.
- Constriction of Chest as if too narrow.
- Painful swollen Glands at sides of neck.
- Soreness high up between the thighs.
- Smarting soreness between the nates.
- The Skin of hands is hard and cracked in several places.
- Finger nails become thick; become black.
- Eruption in the corner of the mouth.
- Itching pimples on the face, become moist after scratching.
- Itching Eruption full of corrosive water in many parts of the body.
- Itching and moist Eruption on scrotum.
- Cracks and Fissure ends of fingers, nipples, labial commissures of anus, between toes, etc.
- Eruption behind ears, oozes a sticky fluid.
- Eczema, with profuse serous exudations; in blondes inclined to obesity.
- Numbness and deadness, with coldness of fingers, extending as far as middle of upper arm.
- Weak exhaustion of whole body.
- Cataleptic conditions; conscious but without power to move or speak.
- Emaciation of suffering parts (Plumb.).

HAMAMELIS VIRGINICA

I. Introduction (Cow.-366)

Synonym: Hamamelis Virginica.
Natural Order: Hamamelaceae.
Common Name: Witch Hazel.
Habitat: A shrub growing in damp woods in USA and Canada.
Preparation: Tincture from the fresh bark of the twigs and roots.

It was first introduced in Homeopathy by Dr. Hoering (Pierce-485).

II. General Analysis (Cow.)

Acts pre-eminently upon the venous system of the blood vessels giving rise to varicosis, haemorrhage and structural legions. Chief expression is passive venous haemorrhage from any part.

III. Suited to (Allen-135)

Veinous haemorrhage from every outlet of the body; nose, lungs, bowels, bladder, uterus. Patients subject to varicose veins; taking cold easily from every exposure, esp. in the warm moist air.

IV. Clinical (Clarke-I-866)

Abortion threatened, Ankles weak, Black-eye, Bruises, Burns, Cancer, Chilblains, Consumption, Enteric fever, Gastric ulcer, Haematemesis, Haematuria, Haemorrhage, Haemorrhagic diathesis, Haemorrhoids, Leucorrhoea, Melaena, Menstruation-abnormal; vicarious, Nipple sore, Noises in head, Nose-bleed, Ovaries-affections of, Pelvic haematocele, Phimosis, Phlegmasia alba dolens, Purpura,

Rheumatism, Scapula-rheumatism of, Scurvy, Small-pox, Testicles inflamed, Ulcer, Uterine affections, Vagina-spasm of, Varicocele, Veins-varicose, Wounds.

V. **Symptoms-General** (Nash-391)

1. Veinous Haemorrhage (very dark and clotted). Veins full, enlarged and sore to touch.

VI. **Symptoms-Particular** (Nash-391)

1. Varicocities of almost every kind (full dilated veins).
   Ham.,
   Fluor. ac.,
   Puls.
2. Soreness as if bruised.
   Ham.-sometimes in Rheumatism succeeded when Arn. failed. Ham. acts upon nose, on veins which are full, enlarged and sore.
   Arn.-more upon capillaries, causing their relaxation, where by suggilation takes place.
3. Haemorrhage-severe bleeding of very dark, clotted and veinous blood from nose, bowels, lungs, uterus, bladder, anus, etc.
4. Orchitis and inflammation of spermatic veins (inflammation of testes).

HELLEBORUS NIGER

I. Introduction (Cow.-369)

Synonym: Helleborus Niger.
Natural Order: Ranunculaceae.
Common Name: Black Hellebore, Christmas Rose.
Habitat: A plant in the mountainous and temperate regions of Europe.
Preparation: Tincture from the dried root.

It was first proved by Hahnemann recording 285 symptoms (Pierce-487).

II. General Analysis (Cow.)

Acts upon kidney (scanty urine), Serous membranes (dropsical affection of the brain, thorax, peritoneum, etc.), Inflammation of stomach and intestines. Through pneumogastric nerves Cardiac paralysis. Chief use is in treatment of hydrocephalus when serous affection has commenced.

III. Suited to (Allen-136)

Weakly, delicate, Psoric children, prone to brain troubles (Bell., Calc. c., Tuberc.), with serous effusion. Irritable, easily angered, consolation <(Ign., Nat. m., Sep., Sil.); does not want to be disturbed (Gels., Nat. m.) stupid (Chronic of Baryt. c.). Melancholy, despairing, silent; in girls at puberty when menses do not return after appearing.

IV. Clinical (Clarke-I-870)

Albuminuria, Amenorrhoea, Aphthae, Apoplexy, Cholera, Concussions, Convulsions, Cystitis, Depression of spirits, Diarrhoea, Dropsy, Epilepsy, Headache, Hernia, Homesickness, Hydrocele, Hydrocephalus, Kidneys-congestion of, Melancholia, Meningitis, Night-blindness, Puerperal convulsions, Scarlatina, Tetanus, Typhoid fever, Ulcer, Wounds.

V. Symptoms-Particular (Nash-264-265)

1. Meningitis-or brain trouble when threatened affection or affection already there.
2. Head rolling side to side on the pillow with screams, one arm and one leg moves, while other one as if paralysed. Great stupidity or soporous sleep, greedy drinking of water, wrinkled forehead, cold sweat; motion of jaws as if chewing; dilated pupils, often can't be made to see or hear or to be made to sense anything at all.
3. Urine scanty or entirely suppressed. Coffee ground sediments in urine.
4. Post Scarlatina dropsy.

   Apis.,
   Hell. n.,
   Hep. s. (278).

HEPAR SULPHURIS

I. Introduction (Cow.-373)

Synonym: Hepar sulfuris Calcaream.
Preparation: Trituration (Impure calcium sulphide).

It was proved by Hahnemann in MMP (with 295 symptoms-3rd Ed.) (Pierce-492).

II. General Analysis

Allen says that Hep. s. simulates Mercury in its action upon liver and kidney; Sul. upon skin and mucous membranes of intestinal tracts; Calcarea upon respiratory tract. Most essential feature-tendency to promote suppuration.

III. Suited to (Allen-139)

Torpid lymphatic constitutions, persons with light hair and complexion; slow to act, muscles soft and flabby. Slightest injury causes suppuration (Graph., Merc. c.). Over sensitive mentally and physically; can't bear uncovering in even hot weather (Psor.) (Nux. v.-Can't cover, Camph., Sec.). Extremely sensitive to cold air. Skin-very sensitive.

IV. Clinical (Clarke-I-894)

Abscess, Amaurosis, Angina pectoris, Appetite disordered, Asthma, Axilla-abscess in, Beard-eruptions of, Blepharitis, Boils, Breast-affections of, Bronchitis, Bubo, Burns, Carbuncles, Caries, Chilblains, Chlorosis, Colds, Constipation, Consumption, Cornea-ulceration of; opacity of, Cough, Croup, Diaphragmitis, Diarrhoea, Ear affections ; polypi of, Eczema, Emphysema, Erysipelas, Eye affections, Fester-tendency to, Glandular swellings, Haemoptysis, Haemorrhoids, Headache, Hectic, Herpes preputialis, Hip-joint disease, Hoarseness, Jaundice, Joint affections,

Laryngitis, Leucorrhoea, Lips swollen, Liver-affections of, Lung affections, Lupus, Marasmus, Menorrhagia, Mouth sore, Nipple sore, Ovaries-affections of, Parametritis, Pleurisy, Pneumonia, Pregnancy-sickness of, Pruritus mercurialis, Pylorus-affections of, Quinsy, Rhagades, Rheumatism, Scarlatina, Scrofula, Skin-affections of, Spinal irritation, Styes, Suppuration, Syphilis, Tenesmus, Throat sore, Urticaria, Wens, Whitlow, Whooping-cough.

V. Symptoms-General (Nash-276)

1. Hypersensitive to touch, pain, cold air; fainting with the pain.
2. General tendency to suppurations; even slight injuries or scratches in the skin suppurate.
3. Tendency to croupy exudations-(Larynx and kidneys; any mucous membrane).
4. Atony; stools passed with great difficulty, even when soft. Urine flows slowly, must wait for it, then drops vertically down without force.
5. Sour diarrhoea; whole child smells sour.
6. Coughs; croup, bronchitis, consumption, <when exposed to least cold air.
7. Modalities; < exposure to dry cold air, > in moist, wet weather.
8. Like Sul., Hep. s. is adapted to the Psoric, scrofulous diathesis.

VI. Symptoms-Particular (Nash-277-82)

1. Great anti Psoric-Stands half way between Sul.-Calc. c.

   Hep. s.,
   Sul.,
   Calc. c.

2. Hypersensitive—to Touch, pain, cold air-It is mental as well as physical, for slightest cause irritates to hasty speech with vehemence.

   China. -to slight touch but can bear hard pressure.
   Ars. - < cold

Calc. c.-< cold
Hep. s. -< cold (Skin sensitive to touch)
Nux. v. -< cold
Psor. -< cold
Sil. -< cold
Tuberc. -< cold

3. Slightest injury suppurates (pus) Where pus is about to be formed or formed.
   Hep. s.-given high before pus to abort; low to hasten suppuration.
   Graph.,
   Merc. c.,
   Petr.
4. Chronic Cold Catarrh-Nose stopped every time he went into cold air.
   Tuberc.-with fresh air gets new cold every time. In warm room feels better.
   Croup-cough-least breath of cold air, loose expectoration but can't raise it, with rattle, comes in the early hours of the morning. After Acon. and Spon. mostly.
   Acon.-Croup after sleep in the evening hours. } brought on by exposure to dry cold air.
   Hep. s.-early morning hours. } brought on by exposure to dry cold air.
5. Chronic Asthma (279).
   Hep. s.-Better in wet/damp weather and worse in dry cold.
   Nat. s.-Worse in wet/damp weather and better in dry cold (Dulc.).
6. Cough when any part is uncovered-Whole case aggravated.
   Hep. s.,
   Baryt. c.,
   Rhus t. (Best after skin affection).
7. Throat-Sticking in, as if splinter or fishbone on swallowing/yawning-extending to the ear.
8. Continuous fish bone sensation-
   Hep. s.,
   Arg. n.,

Dolichos.,
Nit. ac.

9. Quinsy (Acute inflammation of Tonsil).

Bell. -High fever, swelling, redness, headache, throbbing carotids.

Merc. v. -either side, foetid breath, flabby moist intended tongue, sweat without relief.

Lach. -< sleep, left side extending to right, sensitiveness to touch.

Lyc. -Right to left, tongue swollen inclined to protrude, stuffing of nose.

Lac can. -alternates sides every day.

Hep. s. -throbbing pain, chronic hypertrophy of tonsils with hardness of hearing.

Baryt. c.,
Plumb.

10. Stomach longing for Acid things, chronic dyspepsia.

Hep. s.,
Verat..

11. Sour Diarrhoea.

Hep. s.-whole child smells sour.
Mag. c.,
Calc. c. (Even soft stool passed with great difficulty)

} sour stool.

12. Urine-has to wait a while, inability to expel, never able to finish sensation. Some urine always remained behind in bladder feeling. Urine drops vertically without force.

Alumina,
Verat.,
Sil.,
Hep. s.

13. Sweats day and night without relief (in rheumatism).

Hep. s.,
Merc. c. (follows well after Merc. c.-when no relief from sweats).

VII. Black Letter Symptoms

(Tyler-405-7)

- Constant pressive pain in one half of brain as from a plug or nail (Thuj.).
- Epistaxis (Vipera. etc.).
- Great swelling of the upper hip.
- Sticking in throat as from a splinter on swallowing, extending towards the ear on yawning.
- Great desire for vinegar.
- Nausea.
- Abdomen distended, tense.
- Buboes, abscesses of inguinal glands.
- Stool soft, yet passed with great exertion.
- Clay coloured stool.
- Urging to stool but large intestines are wanting in peristaltic action, and can't expel the faeces which are not hard; only a portion of which can be forced out by help of abdominal muscles.
- Very difficult passage of scanty, not hard, faeces, with much urging.
- Micturition impeded; obliged to wait before the urine passes, and then it flows slowly.
- He is never able to finish urinating; it seems as if some urine always remains behind in bladder.
- Slackness of bladder; urine drops vertically down, and he is obliged to wait a while before any passes.
- Paroxysms of cough, as from taking cold, with excessive sensitiveness of the nervous system, as soon as only the slightest portion of the body becomes cold.
- Dyspnoea.
- Abscess of axillary glands.
- Bruised pain in anterior muscles of thigh.
- Swelling of knee.
- Drawing pain in limbs.
- Cracked lines and chaps in hands and feet.
- The ulcer bleeds on being merely gently wiped.
- Eroding pain in ulcer.

- Sensitiveness to open air.
- At night the pains are worst.
- Dreams of fire.
- Night sweat.
- Unhealthy, suppurating skin, even slight injuries maturate and suppurate.
- Soreness and moisture in folds between scrotum and thigh.
- Perspires easily on every, even slight motion.
- Catarrhal fever with great sensitiveness of skin to touch, and to the slightest cold.
- Constant offensive exhalations from the body.
- Among Hahnemann's symptoms are these other peculiar ones which may prove diagnostic.
- The slightest thing put him into a violent passion, and he could have murdered anyone without hesitation.
- Cross; and had such weakness of memory that he required three or four minutes to remember anything, and when at work thoughts often left him all at once.
- In the evening frightful anxiety; thought he must be ruined, and was sad to a degree that he could have killed himself.
- In the morning after waking, he had visionary appearance of a deceased person, which frightened him; also imagined he saw a neighbouring house in flames, which terrified him.
- When the smallest member becomes cool, there immediately occurs a cough, as from a chill and oversensitiveness of nervous system.
- Suffocative cough, excited by tightness of breath.
- At night, from 11 to 12, violent cough.
- Before midnight he sprang out of sleep, full of anxiety, called for help, left he could not get his breath. (Hep. s. is one of the great Croup medicines).
- Even small wounds and slight injuries suppurate, will not heal, and become ulcers.
- Hahnemann says; "Belladonna removes many of the sufferings caused by Hep. s., where the symptoms correspond."

HYDRASTIS CANADENSIS

I. Introduction (Cow.-379)

Synonym: Hydrastis Canadensis.
Natural Order: Ranunculaceae.
Common Name: Golden seal, Orange Rost.
Habitat: A small herbaceous perennial plant in rich wood in Northern and Western USA.
Preparation: Tincture from fresh roots.

Dr. Hale was the first to detect its use in homeopathy (Pierce-498).

II. General Analysis (Cow.)

Acts prominently upon mucous membrane especially of outlets of body eyes, nose, urinary organs etc. Natural secretion increases, then turns to yellow; thick green, even bloody. Then mucous membrane becomes dry and its function is destroyed. It causes-Erythema, moist eruption, eczema ulceration with long of debility either local or general system. Causes Hepatitis, Jaundice, Catarrhal dyspepsia and constipation.

III. Suited to (Allen-142)

Debilitated persons with viscid mucous discharges.

IV. Clinical (Clarke-I-919)

Alcoholism, Asthma, Cancer, Catarrh, Chancroids, Constipation, Corns, Dyspepsia, Eczema impetiginoides, Ear affections, Faintness, Fistula, Gastric catarrh, Gonorrhoea, Haemorrhoids, Jaundice, Leucorrhoea, Lip-cancer of, Liver-affections of, Lumbago, Lupus, Menorrhagia, Metrorrhagia, Mouth sore, Nails-affections of, Nipple sore, Noises in head, Nursing women-sore mouth of, Ozaena, Placenta-adherent, Post-nasal catarrh, Rectum-affections of, Sciatica, Seborrhoea, Stomach-affections of, Syphilis, Taste disordered, Throat-deafness, Throat sore, Tongue-affections of, Typhus, Ulcer, Uterus-affections of.

V. Symptoms-General (Nash-397)

1. Pain and very weak, faint, gone feeling in stomach, which is sometimes actually sunken.
2. Affections of the mucous membranes, where there is a viscid stringy discharge; stomach, bronchi, uterus, etc.
3. Chronic constipation is remarkable for its absence of any other symptom.

VI. Symptoms-Particular (Nash-398)

1. Dull aching pain in the stomach which causes a very weak, faint, gone feeling in epigastrium.
   Sep.-with uterine affections.
   Ign.-purely nervous reasons.
2. Chronic constipation-Infantile constipation.
3. Affections of Mucous membrane with viscid, stringy discharge (Kali. bich.). Also-chronic bronchi-Leucorrhoea.

HYOSCYAMUS NIGER

I. Introduction (Cow.-384)

Synonym: Hyoscyamus Niger.
Natural Order: Solanaceae.
Common Name: Henbane.
Habitat: A plant native of Europe. Grows on rubbish.
Preparation: Tincture from fresh plant.

It was first proved by Hahnemann (580 symptoms in MMP) (Pierce-504).

II. General Analysis (Cow.)

Acts esp. upon cerebro-spinal system affecting sensorium and muscular system. In former causing hallucinations, illusions, distinct mania bordering quarrelsome or obscure character. Its functional excitement is moderate. On muscular system it produces paralysis of involuntary system, spasmodic affections of single parts. Chief activity-sensorial activity and nervous excitement.

III. Suited to (Allen-142)

Sanguine temperament, irritable, nervous, hysterical. Convulsion-child from fright, from worms (Cina.); during labour, child-sudden shriek, then insensible. Disease with increased cerebral activity but non-inflammatory. Cough-< night-after eating-drinking talking, singing, (Dros., Phos.-> lying down, Mang.). Intense sleeplessness-business problems-imaginary. Bladder-Paralysis after labour with retention or incontinence; no desire to urinate in lying in women (Arn., Op.). Involuntary Stool/Urine.

IV. Clinical (Clarke-I-940)

Amaurosis, Angina pectoris, Bladder-paralysis of, Bronchitis, Chorea, Coma vigil, Cough, Delirium tremens, Diarrhoea,

Dysmenorrhoea, Enteric fever, Epilepsy, Epistaxis, Erotomania, Eye affections, Haemoptysis, Haemorrhage, Hiccough, Hydrophobia, Hypochon-driasis, Lochia suppressed, Mania, Meningitis, Mind-affections of, Neuralgia, Night-blindness, Nymphomania, Paralysis, Paralysis agitans, Parotitis, Pneumonia, Puerperal mania, Rage, Sleep disordered, Stammering, Tetanus, Toothache, Urine-retention of, Vision disordered.

V. **Symptoms-General** (Nash-105)

1. High grade delirium, similar to that of Stram. and Bell.: alternating with low-grade delirium, with stupor, equal to that of Opium. Face pale.
2. Grasping at flocks, picking the bed clothes and subsultus tendium (Twitching of tendons and muscles, especially around wrists).
3. Persistent cough, worse lying down. Relieved on sitting up, especially in elderly people.
4. Dementia senilis; fears imaginary things, being poisoned, sees persons and things that are not present; foolish laughter.
5. General twitching of all the muscles of the body; in spasms or Convulsion.
6. The mania often takes on the lascivious from. The patient uncovers and exposes himself, sings and talks amorously.
7. Fears being poisoned; suspicious and jealous.
8. Constant staring at surrounding objects, self-forgetful (Fever), Pupils dilated; insensible, small objects seem very large, Sordes on teeth; grating the teeth. Alternates well with Rhus t. (Fever).

VI. **Symptoms-Particular** (Nash-106-8)

1. Delirium Trio-Bell., Hyo., Stram.

   Bell. -Violent form predominates, red face, head remedy.

   Hyo. -Stupid muttering predominates with.
   -Occassional violence.
   -Face pale

-Weakness (Not so much as in Bell. or Stram.) and weakness increases.

-Gradually goes to unconsciousness (Op.) with eyes open.

-Stool etc. pass involuntarily (leading in *Typhoid*).

-High graded alternates with low.

2. Chronic Mania-(acute delirium into settled from).
   a. Suspicious (Hyo. best) someone plotting to poison him, jealous of others. Jealous. Lascivious. (Hyo. is leader).
   b. Weak-due to infirmity of age (suited to as well).
3. Twitching of every muscle; twitch in the entire body-Eye to Toe.

   -Not tonic but of clonic order as in Nux. v., Strych.

   -Not so violent as under Cic. v.
4. Cough Dry < when lying, > better when sitting, worse Lying esp. old.
5. Scarlatina Typhoid-Hyo. alternates with Rhus t. when Rhus t. does not clear depression (only alternation Nash says he is guilty of-Pg.-108).

VII. Black Letter Symptoms (Tyler-413-414)

- Ravings: delirium: with restlessness: would not stay in bed.
- Foolish laughter: talks more than usual: more animatedly: hurriedly.
- Silly: smiling: laughs at everything: silly expression.
- Comical alienation of mind: performs ludicrous actions like monkeys.
- Makes ridiculous gestures like a dancing clown.
- Strips himself naked: lies in bed and prattles.
- Carphology. Picks at bedclothes: mutters and prattles.
- Unable to think: cannot direct or control thoughts.
- Answers no questions: cannot bear to be talked to.
- Is violent, and beats people.
- Jealousy with rage and delirium: with attempt to murder.
- Lascivious mania; uncovers; sings amorous songs.

- Suspicious Fears; alone; of being poisoned (Lach., Rhus t., etc.), of being injured. Wants to run away. Fears being bitten.
- Wants to get up and attend to business, or go home (Bry.).
- Delirium; talks of business; of imaginary wrongs.
- Pupils dilated; insensible.
- Small objects seem very large (reverse of Plat.).
- Constant starting at surrounding objects. Self-forgetful.
- Pressive squeezing on the root of the Nose.
- Deafness (from paralysis of auditory nerve).
- Swallowing difficult; inability to swallow.
- Tongue red or brown; dry, cracked, hard, looks like burnt leather, or clean, parched; white, tremulous, Foam at mouth.
- Sordes teeth and mouth, Grating the teeth.
- Dread of water (Stram.).
- Hiccough.
- Inflammation of stomach, or peritonitis with hiccough.
- Cutting low down in the abdomen, pinching in abdomen.
- Urging to stool. Stool passed involuntarily in bed.
- No will to make water in childbed.
- Puerperal spasms; shrieks; anguish; chest oppressed; unconscious.
- Much mucous in larynx and air passages, which makes voice and speech not clear.
- Almost incessant cough while lying down; disappears when sitting up. Dry cough at night.
- Cough at night; frequent cough at night. Which always wakes him, after which he again falls asleep.
- Angular motions; jerks of single muscles or sets of muscles.
- Subsultus tendinum.
- Convulsion;
- Suffocating spells and Convulsion during labour.
- Epilepsy. Before attack-vertigo, sparks before eyes, ringing in ears, hungry gnawing; during attack-face

purple, eyes projecting shrinks, grinds teeth, urination.

- Epileptoid spasms, Epilepsy daily so violent it seemed as if spine or joints would be broken.
- Very profound slumber.
- Sleeplessness; long-continued sleeplessness; on account of quiet mental activity.
- Unable to sleep the whole night; tried lying on one side and the other; yet unable to get quiet (Ars.).
- Starts from sleep as if in a fright.
- Intense sleeplessness of irritable, excitable persons from business embarrassments-often imaginary.
- Sleepless, or constant sleep, with muttering.
- Long continued sleeplessness.
- Can't bear to be talked to, or least noise during chill.

IGNATIA

I. Introduction (Cow.-390)

Synonym: Strychnos Ignatia.
Natural Order: Logainaceae.
Common Name: St. Ignatius Bean.
Habitat: A large shrub or small tree in Cochine-China and Philippines.
Preparation: Tincture or trituration from powdered seeds.

It was first proved by Hahnemann (Pierce-509).

II. General Analysis (Cow.)

Primary action upon oblongata and nervous system giving tetanic convulsion and dyspnoea-secondary action upon entire nervous system giving increased susceptibility to external impressions, both mental and physical. Convulsive twitching and spasms, or these alternating with torpor and depression. The leading expression is finely sensitive mood, with sadness and silent grief and constantly brooding over imaginary troubles.

III. Suited to (Allen-145)

Nervous temperament, esp. women of sensitive, easily excitable nature, dark hair and skin, but mild, quick to perceive, rapid in execution. Show of indecision (Puls.). Easily offended. Striking contrast to Puls. Long, continued grief.

IV. Clinical (Clarke-II-6)

Abdomen distended, Anger-effects of, Anus-affections of, Anxiety, Appetite disordered, Back-weakness of, Catalepsy, Change of life, Chorea, Clavus, Convulsions, Croup, Debility, Dentition, Depression of spirits, Diphtheria, Dysmenorrhoea, Epilepsy, Fainting, Fear-effects of, Flatulence-obstructed, Glands enlarged, Haemorrhoids, Headache, Heart affections, Hiccough, Hysteria, Hysterical joint, Intermittent fever, Locomotor ataxy, Melancholia, Numbness, Oesophagus, Paralysis, Phlyctenular ophthalmia, Proctalgia, Rectum-prolapse of, Rheumatic fever, Sciatica, Sensitiveness, Sinking, Sleep disordered, Spinal irritation, Tenesmus, Throat sore, Toothache, Tremors, Urine abnormal, Vagina-spasm of, Voice lost, Yawning.

V. Symptoms-General (Nash-163)

1. Remedy of paradoxicalities. Head better lying on painful side, moody, gonencess > not by eating, sore throat < by swallowing. Thirst during chill, face red during chill, etc.
2. Sad, sighing, changeable, moody disposition.
3. Twitching or spasms, or convulsion from exciting or depressing emotions, fright, etc.
4. All gone, weak, empty sensation in stomach not > by eating.
5. Anal troubles (Piles, prolapsus, soreness and pain shooting up into abdomen.).
6. Adapted to emotional hysterical subjects.
7. Modalities; < slight touch, smoking, coffee; > lying on painful side; hard pressure; profuse watery urination.
8. Cough; dry, spasmodic; not relieved by coughing, the longer he coughs the more the irritation to cough increases.
9. Pain; in small circumscribed spots; over-sensitive (Coff., Hep. s.).
10. In most cases Ignatia should be given in the morning. Ignatia bears the same relation to the diseases of women that Nux. v. does to bilious men.

VI. Symptoms-Particular (Nash-164-170)

1. Mental Medicine (nervous) with marked element of Sadness. Sad, Sighing.

   (Ign. = Female, Nux. v. = bilious male).

   Acon.,

Cham.,
Nux. v.,
Coff.,
Hep. s. (Sensitive to touch).
Ign.-marked sadness, deep breaths, silent suffering, tries to hide that.
grief from others.

2. Changeable Moods-No remedy can equal Ign.
   (a) Ign. hysterical affections. Changeability in greatest degree-full of glee at one moment, sad with tears suddenly. Again impatient, quarrelsome, angry mood (not to Cham. degree).
   Acon.,
   Coff.,
   Nux. m.,
   (b) Effects of Fright-Acon.
   (c) Quarrelsome. angry mood.
   Cham.,
   Ign.-not to the degree of Cham.
   Op.
   Verat.,
3. Nervous; Convulsion, Twitchings all over body (Chorea) spasmodic affection originating in mental causes, as after fright, punishment of children etc.
   Ign.-also in paralysis with hysteria, Long drawn sighs (indicator).
   Nux. v.,
   Zinc.-closest to Ign. in symptoms.
   Agar.,
   Cupr.,
   Hyo.
   Verat. v.
4. Over sensitive to pain.
   Ign.,
   Acon.,
   Coff.,
   Cham.
5. Headache as if nail driven and with changeable symptoms.
   Ign.

(a) Nervous, hysterical; One sided headache > lying on painful.

side > lying on it.

(b) Sometimes-comes on gradually, abates suddenly-Sul. ac.,

-comes on suddenly, abates suddenly-Bell.

Nux. v.-for men } nervous, changeableness of symptoms is most prominent in headaches.
Ign.-for women }

(c) Profuse urine releaves (Headache esp. in nervous women).

Acon.,
Gels.,
Sil.,
Verat.,
Lac def. (profuse flow during headache).

(d) Headache < by coffee/smoking/Alcohol/close attention/pressing at stool/close attention, snuff, tobacco smoke,

> eating (Psor.) but soon after.

< Cold wind, light, noise, sudden turning of head, stooping.

looking up long, moving eyes.

> Soft pressive external heat, profuse urine, warmth.

6. Pain in throat relieved by swallowing < between acts of deglutition. Globus Hystericus-as if a lump came up from stomach to throat (Caps.) as if to choke, but is swallowed down, but comes up again.

Ign.-Better from solid swallowing < from liquid swallowing.

Bap.-Can swallow liquid only, least food gags.

Lach.-Like Ign.

7. Empty gone feeling at the pit of stomach, with sigh or to take deep breath.

Ign.-with sigh or long breath, sometimes feeling as if stomach hung down relaxed.

Hydras., -goneness in the stomach.
Sep.,

Ipec.-as if stomach hangs down relaxed.

Gastralgia of hysterical women, Ign. is first remedy to be thought of.

8. Anal Rectal symptoms-Frequent desire for stool.
   Nux. v.-Frequent desire, very little stool. But in Ign. in place of stool, comes out prolapsed rectum.
   Ign. -rectum prolapsus, sharp shooting pain upwards in rectum (Sep.-similar pain in uterus).
   Nit. ac.-Pain after loose and soft stool.
   Rut. -Rectum Prolapse-like Ign.
   Sep. -sharp shooting pains.
9. Fever-Intermittant-Ign. is a unique remedy for (Nash-169).
   Ign. -thirst during chill and in no other stage. Ign. is only.
   remedy with this symptom.
   -Chill relieved by heat external.
   -Heat aggravated by external covering (Nux. v.-reverse).
   -Red face during chill.
   Caps. -Chill between shoulders.
   Eup. perf.-Chill in AM, Bone pain and vomit after chill.
   Smoke of tobacco-extreme aversion to-in many complaints (168).

VII. Black Letter Symptoms (Tyler-429-31)

- Uncommon tendency to be frightened.
- Audacity.
- Fickle, impatient, irresolute, quarrelsome, recurring every 3 to 4 hours.
- Incredible changes of disposition, at one time he jokes and jests, at another he is lachrymose, alternately every three to four hours.
- Whispering voice. He can't speak loudly.
- Delicate disposition, with very clear consciousness.
- Finely sensitive mood, delicate conscientiousness.
- Slight blame or contradiction excites him to anger and this makes him angry with himself.
- Incredible changes of mood.

- Heat in the head, head is heavy.
- He hangs the head forward, Lays the head forward on the table.
- Headache, increased by stooping forwards.
- Aching pain in forehead above root of nose which compels him to bend forward the head, followed by inclination to vomit.
- Headache like a pressure with something hard on the surface of the brain, recurring in fits.
- Throbbing headache, Headache at every beat of the arteries.
- Itching in the auditory meatus.
- Shooting in the lips.
- Inner surface of lower lip painful, as if raw and excoriated.
- Lips are cracked and bleed.
- He is apt to bite on one side of the tongue posteriorly when speaking or chewing.
- Stitches in palate extending into the external ear.
- Sour taste in the mouth.
- Aching pain in cervical glands.
- Formication in the oesophagus.
- Belches up a bitter fluid.
- What he has ingested is belched up again into the mouth.
- Retching (Constrictive) sensation in the middle of the throat as if there were a large morsel of food or a plug sticking there, felt more when not swallowing than when swallowing.
- Sore throat; sticking in it when not swallowing and even somewhat while swallowing; the more he swallows, the more it disappears; if he swallows anything solid, like bread, it seems as though the sticking entirely disappeared.
- After eating and drinking, hiccough.
- Aching in scrobiculus cordis.
- Extreme aversion to smoking tobacco.
- A feeling in the stomach as from fasting.
- Feeling of flabbiness in the stomach.
- Peculiar sensation of weakness in upper abdomen and pit of stomach, and paleness of face.

- Rumbling and rattling in the bowels.
- On the left, above the navel, a sharp shooting.
- Pinching and shooting pains in abdomen.
- Prolapsus of the rectum during moderate straining at stool.
- Violent urging to stool, more in the upper bowels and upper part of the abdomen. He has great desire, yet the stool, though soft, does not pass in sufficient quantity.
- Painless contraction of the anus.
- A coarse stitch from anus deep into rectum.
- Pain one or two hours after stool, pain in rectum, as from blind piles compounded of contraction and sore pain.
- Blind piles, painful while sitting and standing, less while walking.
- Prolapsus of the rectum, from moderate exertion at stool.
- Sharp pressive pain in the rectum.
- Sore pain in the anus, without reference to the stool.
- Great urgency and desire for stool in the evening, felt mostly in the middle of the abdomen, but no stool follows, only the rectum protrudes.
- Frequent discharge of much watery urine.
- Irritation and ulcerative pain-genitalia.
- Complete absence of sexual desire, alternating with the reverse.
- Provocation to cough in larynx, not relieved by cough, but only by suppressing cough.
- Sensation of dry feathery dust in pit of throat, not relieved by coughing; but more excited the more he allow himself to cough. Inspiration is impeded as by a weight lying upon him; expiration is all the easier.
- Single jerking of the limbs, on falling asleep.
- Pain in sacrum, also when lying on the back in the morning in bed.
- Pain in the joint of the humerus when bending the arm back, as from prolonged hard work, or as if bruised.
- In the deltoid muscle a quivering twitching.

- Hot knees with cold nose.
- Creeping, gone-to-sleep feeling of the limbs.
- In the joints of the shoulders, hip and knees, a pain as from a sprain or dislocation.
- Simple violent pain, only felt when touched here and there on a small spot, e.g. on the ribs, etc.
- Sleep so light that he hears everything in it.
- Snoring inspiration during sleep.
- Fixed idea in dream, Dreamed all night of the same subject.
- One ear and one cheek red and burning.
- Sudden attack of flying heat all over the body.
- External heat and redness, without internal heat.
- External warmth is intolerable.
- Feeling as if sweat would break out.
- Shaking chill with redness of the face.

IODIUM

I. Introduction (Cow.-397)

Common Name: Iodine.
Preparation: One part by weight of resumblimed Iodine, dissolved in 99 parts by weight of Alcohol-makes 2x dilution.

It was introduced to homeopathy by Hahnemann (Pierce-515).

II. General Analysis (Cow.)

Affects every organ and tissue of the body but especially the lymphatic glands and mucous tissues, having depressing and atonizing influence with general emaciation. The glandular action is notably upon the thyroid, the mesenteric, the mammae, ovaries, and testicles, on the mucous membranes of the eyes, nose and entire respiratory tract with high temperature, lungs. Sometimes a catarrhal inflammation is produced. Chief expression-Local and general emaciation with typical iodine conditions.

III. Suited to (Allen-148)

Persons of scrofulous (tuberculous) diathesis with black dark hair and eyes, a low cachectic condition with profound debility and emaciation (Abrot.), great weakness and loss of breath going upstairs (Calc. c.); during menses (Alumina, Cocc.).

IV. Clinical (Clarke-II-27)

Appetite disordered, Atrophy, Brain-atrophy of, Breasts-affection of, Cancer, Chilblains, Chyluria, Constipation, Consumption, Coryza, Cough, Croup, Debility, Diabetes, Diarrhoea, Diphtheria, Emaciation, Enteric fever, Galactorrhoea, Goitre, Haemorrhoids, Headaches, Heart-hypertrophy of; affections of, Hiccough, Hydrocephalus, Iritis, Jaundice,

Joint affections, Lactation disordered, Laryngitis, Leucorrhoea, Liver-affections of, Lymphatic swellings, Melancholia, Mollities ossium, Ovaries-affection of; dropsy of, Ozaena, Prostate enlarged, Rheumatic gout, Rheumatism, Salivation, Scars, Seborrhoea, Sterility, Syphilis, Tabes mesenterica, Throat-affections of, Uterine affections, Voice-affections of, Vomiting, Worms.

V. Symptoms-General (Nash-354)

1. Always hungry, eats or wants to, all the time, yet emaciates, > while eating.
2. Hypertrophy of all glands except mammary, which dwindle; while body withers, glands enlarge.
3. Mentally; anguish, wants to move, do something, hurry, kill somebody, etc. (Ars.).
4. Warm blooded not withstanding emaciation, wants a cool place to move, think or work in.
5. Pulsations all over; stomach, back, even arms, fingers and toes (Bell.).
6. Especially suited to dark-haired, dark-eyed, dark-skinned persons of scrofulous habit.
7. Modalities; < fasting, in warm air or room, > while eating moving, and cold air.
8. Great weakness and loss of breath on going up stairs.
9. Hard goitre in dark-haired persons; also tumours in the breast.
10. Sensation as if the heart was squeezed together; as if grasped with an iron hand (Sul.).
11. Croup; membranous; in scrofulous children. Child grasps the larynx; face pale and cold; in fleshy children.

VI. Symptoms-Particular (Nash-355)

Anti-scrofulous remedy.

1. Scrofulous diathesis, cachectic condition with profound debility and great emaciation.
2. Remarkable and unaccountable sense of weakness and loss of breath on going up stairs.
3. Ravenous hunger; eats often, and much, but loses

flesh > after eating or while eating, progressive emaciation.

4. Dwindling of mammae and soreness.
5. Profuse uterine haemorrhage, Cancer of uterus.
6. Chronic leucorrhoea, abundant and so corrosive as to eat holes in the liver.
7. Swelling of glands, esp. mesenteric (middle of intestine) and thyroid.
8. Membranous croup, wheezing, sawing, respiration dry, barking cough, especially in children with dark eyes and hairs, child grasps the throat when coughing.
9. < Warm room in general.

VII. Black Letter Symptoms (Tyler-432-33)

- Staring with wide open eyes, lids seem to retracted.
- Nasal catarrh thin, excoriating.
- Increase of saliva; mercurial salivation.
- Suffers from hunger, must eat every few hours; gets anxious and worried if he eats; feels better after eating.
- Ravenous hunger, can't be satisfied.
- Most symptoms are better after eating.
- Empty Eructation from morning till evening, as if every particle of food turned into "air".
- Left hypochondriac region hard and acutely painful to pressure: Spleen enlarged after intermittent.
- Chronic leucorrhoea, worse at menstrual period, makes thighs sore and corrodes linen.
- Dry cough, with stitches and burning in chest.
- Itching low down in lungs, behind sternum; causing cough; extends through bronchi to nasal cavity.
- Sensation as if Heart were squeezed together, as if heart were grasped by a hand (Lil. t.).
- Palpitation of heart; worse least exertion; with faintness.
- Chronic arthritis, with violent nightly pains in Joints, no swelling.

- Great weakness and loss of breath on going up stairs.
- Hypertrophy and induration of Glands.
- Scrofulous diathesis.
- Low cachectic condition, with profound debility and great emaciation.

IPECACUANHA

I. Introduction (Cow.-402)

Synonym: Cephaelis Ipecacuanha.
Natural Order: Rubiaceae.
Common Name: Ipecac.
Habitat: Small shrub in moist shady woods in Brazil.
Preparation: Tincture from dried root.

It was first proved by Hahnemann (230 symptoms in MMP) (Pierce-519).

II. General Analysis (Cow.)

Acts upon pneumo-gastric nerve, producing spasmodic irritation, mostly in chest, stomach; asthma in the chest and nausea and vomiting in the latter. It irritates mucous membranes of respiratory and digestive tracts causing catarrhal conditions, pulmonary congestion; even haemorrhage from mucous surfaces. Chief expression is—a persistent nausea and vomiting in all diseases.

III. Suited to (Allen-149)

Where gastric symptoms predominate (Ant. c., Puls.) tongue clean or slightly coated. In all diseases with constant and continued nausea. Vomiting of large quantity of mucous without relief (with relief-Ant. tar..).

IV. Clinical (Clarke-II-37)

Anaemia, Asthma, Bronchitis, Catarrh, Cholera, Consumption, Convulsions, Cough, Deafness, Diarrhoea, Dysentery, Enteric fever, Eye affections, Gall-stone colic, Gastric ulcer, Haematemesis, Haemorrhage, Haemorrhoids, Hysteria, Intermittent fever, Menstruation disordered, Opium habit, Pregnancy-affections of, Remittent fever, Salivation, Tetanus, Toothache, Vomiting, Whooping-cough, Worm fever, Yellow fever.

V. Symptoms-General (Nash-228)

1. Persistent nausea, which nothing relieves, in many complaints.
2. Headache as if bruised, all through the bones of the head, down into root of tongue, with nausea.
3. Stools as if fermented, or as green as grass, with colic and nausea.
4. Haemorrhage from uterus; profuse, bright blood and heavy breathing, with nausea.
5. Spasmodic, or asthmatic cough; great depression and wheezing breathing; child becomes rigid and turns blue.
6. Backache, short chill, long fever, heat usually with thirst, raging headache, nausea; and sweat last. Nausea during Pyrexia (feverish).
7. Better than Quinine in intermittents, or after its abuse, the symptoms agreeing.

VI. Symptoms-Particular (Nash-229-235)

1. Nausea, persistent not > after vomiting; from gastric disorder, with clean tongue (Puls.).

    Tongue-clean.

    Ant. c.-(coated).

    Ipec.-Perfect clean tongue or slight coating, effects whole alimentary.

    canal, stomach as if relaxed and hanging down.

    Ipec. stools with.

    vomit, Cholera Infantum or Enterocolitis.

    Puls.-often coated.

    Cina.-worm with clean tongue.

    Dig.-heart trouble with clean tongue.

2. Nothing relieves nausea; face pale, eyes sunken, with blue margin, sleepiness after vomiting, twitching of face and lips.

Ant. tar.- Zinc. s- Lobel.- Apom.-	all powerful emetics, but nausea not so persistent, or found with so many affections.

3. Burning in stomach with thirst, restlessness but can't drink.
   Ipec.,
   Ars.-Often best remedy to follow Ipec. if case goes from bad to worse.
4. Threatened Suffocation from accumulation of Mucous.
   Ipec.-mucous like a foreign body. But Ipec. is often the best when formation of mucous has not begun, i.e. 1st stage, suffocating.
   cough, he becomes stiff and blue in face.
   Ant. tar.-Blue face.
5. Whooping-cough with nose bleed.
   Ipec.-bleeding from mouth, loses breath, turns pale or blue (Indigo).
6. Inflantile Pneumonia. Pale face, body blue; chest loaded with mucous. Rapid and wheezing respiration.
   Comp: Emphysema (distension) of old people.
7. Haemorrhage from all outlet of the body with following:
   Ipec.-Bright red, profuse, heavy breathing (Crot. t-decomposed blood).
   Sul. ac.-Better than Sec. in post partum haemorrhage.
   Acon.-Bright with, fear (great) and anxiety.
   Arn.-from Injury and bodily fatigue, physical exertion.
   Bell.-Blood hot, throbbing carotid, congestion to head.
   Carb. v.-Collapse, to be fanned, pale face.
   China-great loss of blood, ringing in ears, faintness.
   Croc.-Blood clots, in long dark strings.
   Ferr.-partly fluid and solid, Red face or pale alternates.
   Hyo.-Delirium, Jerking and twitching of muscles.
   Lach.-Blood decomposed sediments like charred straw.
   Crot. t., Elap., Sul. ac.-Black fluid Blood, first and last from all outlets.
   Nit. ac.-active, bright Blood, haemorrhage of.
   Phos.-Profuse and persistent bleeding even from small wounds.

Plat.-Partly fluid partly hard clots.
Puls.-Intermittent haemorrhage.
Sec.-Passive flow in women (cachetic, feeble).
Sul.-In Psoric constitution, other remedies fail.

8. Intermittant Fever-in the beginning of all cases (Jahr.).

Ipec.-Persistent Nausea in one or all stages
Ars.-Intense thirst for small quantities during heat, restless, irregularly developed paroxysm.
Eup. perf.-Bone pains, vomits bile at the end of chill, 7-9 AM.
Ign.-> external heat, sighing, chill with red face.
Caps.-chill between shoulder blades and then spreads.
Nux. v.-during heat can't uncover in least, without chill.
Nat. m.-chill 10-11 AM. Headache during chill, sweat >; after quinine.
Rhus t.-Cough in chill, dry Tongue in heat, tossing about; restless.
Podo.-Great loquacity during chill and heat jaundice.
Ant. tar.-great sleepiness during heat and sweat, with pale face.
Remittents also come under the control of this medicine-Ipec.

VII. Black Letter Symptoms (Tyler-444-446)

- Sulky humour, that despises everything, and he desires that others also should not esteem or care for anything.
- Extreme impatience.
- Ailments from vexation and reserved displeasure.
- Headache as if brain and skull were bruised, which penetrates through all the bones of the head down to the root of the tongue, with nausea. Nausea; vomiting; better out of doors.
- Headache as of a bruise of brain and skull, which pierces through all the cranial bones into roots of teeth; with nausea.

- Gastric headaches, occurring in nervous, sensitive persons, commencing with nausea and vomiting.
- Pupils more readily dilatable; dilatation of pupils.
- Eye-gum in the outer canthi of the eyes.
- Nose-bleed, blood, bright red; face pale.
- Profuse accumulation of saliva.
- Nausea as from stomach, with empty Eructation, and great flow of saliva.
- Nausea and vomiting. Distressing nausea.
- Averse to all food. No appetite; earthy taste; stomach feels relaxed; nausea.
- Nausea; distressing; constant, with almost all complaints, with empty Eructation accumulation of much saliva; qualmishness, and efforts to vomit.
- Nausea, with distension of abdomen and dryness in throat; after vomiting inclines to sleep.
- Indescribably sick feeling in stomach.
- Sensation as if stomach hung down relaxed.
- Pain most sever in front of abdomen, extending to left hypochondrium to sides, to back, and base of chest, with swelling of stomach great agitation; constant nausea proceeding from stomach, with empty Eructation and accumulation of much saliva; easy vomiting; diarrhoea.
- Pinching pain in both hypochondria and in the region of pit of stomach.
- Cutting pain about the navel with shivering.
- Distressed feeling in abdomen, as though stomach were hanging down relaxed.
- Griping, as from a hand, each finger sharply pressing into intestines; better during rest, much worse by motion.
- Flatulent colic; about navel as though bowels were grasped by hand.
- Cutting colic near umbilicus; sometimes shivering.
- Tenderness and pain about umbilicus, towards uterus.
- Stools frequent; of greenish mucous.
- Diarrhoeic, and, as it were, fermented, stools.
- Urine cloudy, with sediment like brick dust.
- Dry cough from a tickle in upper part of larynx.

- Cough which arises from a contractive tickling from upper part of larynx to the lowest extremities of the bronchial tubes.
- Rattling in bronchi when drawing a long breath; large accumulation of mucous in bronchi, difficult to raise.
- Rattling noise in air passages during respiration.
- Cough causing inclination to vomit without nausea.
- Suffocating cough, whereby child becomes quite stiff and blue in the face.
- Dyspnoea.
- Difficulty of breathing from least exertion.
- Violent degree of dyspnoea, with wheezing and great weight and anxiety about precordia.
- Spasmodic asthma with great constriction in throat and chest with which a peculiar kind of wheezing nose is heard.
- Loses breath with cough, turns pale and stiffens.
- The body of the child is stretched out stiffly.
- Whooping-cough with nose-bleed; bleeding from mouth; vomiting loses breath, turns pale a blue and becomes rigid.
- Phlegm rattling on chest; sometimes vomited, in young children.
- Haemorrhage from lungs; bright red; coming up with slight effort. < from least exertion; frequent hacking with expectoration of blood-stained mucous; with or without cough; after disturbed catamenia; after mechanical injuries; after former bleedings have weakened lungs; with dry cough in phthisis.
- Pain in all the bones as if bruised.
- Pain in all the joints, as when limbs go to sleep.
- Starts up in sleep.
- Tetanic spasms from swallowing tobacco.
- Fever; backache, short chilling fever, heat usually with thirst, headache, nausea and cough.
- Paroxysms suppressed by quinine.
- Haemorrhage; bright red, from all the orifices of the body; after mechanical injuries.

IRIS VERSICOLOR

I. Introduction (Cow.-406)

Synonym: Iris Hexagona.
Natural Order: Iridaceae.
Common Name: Blue Flag.
Habitat: An indigenous plant found in low wet places, in meadows, and on borders of swamps.
Preparation: Tinctures from the fresh roots.

It was first proved by Dr. JC Rowland in 1852 (Pierce-523).

II. General Analysis (Pierce)

Acts upon glandular and gastro-intestinal mucous membranes causing abnormal activity, increasing secretions to acrid, and causing an increasing flow of bile from the liver, increase flow of urine, on skin vesicular and pustular eruption, gastro-hepatic derangement. Chief characteristic-sick headache from gastro-hepatic derangement.

III. Clinical (Clarke-II-50)

Anus-fissure of, Bilious attack, Constipation, Crusta lactea, Diabetes (pancreatic), Diarrhoea, Dysentery, Dysmenorrhoea, Dyspepsia, Eczema, Fistula, Gastrodynia-intermittent, Headache, Impetigo, Liver-affections of, Migraine, Neuralgia, Nocturnal emissions, Pancreas-affections of, Parotid glands-affections of, Pregnancy-morning sickness of, Psoriasis, Rectum-burning in, Rheumatism, Salivation, Sciatica, Vomiting, Whitlow, Zoster.

IV. Symptoms-General (Nash-237)

1. Burning of mouth, tongue, throat, clear down into stomach, and of anus if there is diarrhoea
2. Vomiting of stringy, glairy, ropy mucous; in strings down to receptacle on the floor.

3. Gastric or hepatic sick headaches with blur before the eyes at the beginning, Vomiting sour, or bitter.

V. Symptoms-Particular (Nash-238)

1. Serviceable in Cholera infantum.
2. Vomit-very sour, Burning, vomit excoriates (scrapes) the throat.
3. Vomit of stringy or ropy mucous mouth to floor, vomit becomes coffee ground like colour. Effective when Kali bich. failed.
4. Sick Headache. Of gastric, hepatic origin with a blur before the eyes.
5. Gastric trouble-Often accompanied with burning of tongue, throat, oesophagus and stomach, if diarrhoea present, then of anus. This entire burning in the alimentary canal is very characteristic of this medicine.

VI. Black Letter Symptoms (Tyler-450)

- Sick Headache, of gastric or hepatic origin, always beginning with a blur before eyes.
- Dull throbbing or shooting, right forehead; nausea.
- Worse; evening, rest, cold air, coughing.
- Better from moderate motion.
- Sharp cutting pains of short duration, changing often.
- Mouth and tongue feel as though scalded.
- Profuse flow of saliva.
- Nausea and Vomiting: of sour food, whole persons smells sour; of thin, watery fluid of exceedingly sour taste.
- Watery STOOL, Anus feels on fire; disposition to strain and bear down; great burning in anus.
- Anus feels sore; severe burning in anus after stool.
- Anus feels sore, or as if sharp points were sticking in it.
- HERPES zoster on right side of body.

KALI SALTS

(Pierce-526-28)

Among alkalis, Allen says, Kali salts are the most poisonous. They are very complex in nature since they produce divergent alternation of both function and nutrition.

They produce profound anaemia, increasing all secretions, especially the quantity of urine, while at the same time elimination of solid constituents, such as uric acid and urea, is increased.

- Kidney becomes inflamed and degenerates.
- Digestion becomes impaired because the alkaline stomach does not favour accumulation of food.
- Patient is always tired and cold.
- Paralysis of heart-cardiac depression, not cardiac failure, as these salts affect other nerves, not the pneumo-gastric nerves.

Essential features of Potash disease are

- Emaciation.
- Excessive waste in secretions.
- Anaemia.
- a low, feeble pulse threatening cardiac failure.

Negative points are

- Absence of fever.
- No excitement.

While selecting a Potash salt special attention must be paid to

1. Character of secretions in mucous membranes.
2. Character of pains.
3. Period of aggravation.

Potash salts are far more poisonous then Soda salts.

KALI BROMATUM

I. Introduction (Cow-415)

Common Name: Bromide of Potash.
Preparation: Centicimal Scale and Triturations.

It was proved by Dr. Hoering and Hermerdinger of Germany in 1838 (Pierce-534).

II. General Analysis (Cow.)

Acts upon nervous system and nerve centres, intellectual weakness, loss of memory, of words, anaesthesia of skin, melancholia, mucous membranes of eye, throat; loss of sexual power, boils, imbecility. Functional paralysis of nearly all organs of the body and tissues, acne-like Eruption, especially upon face, neck and shoulders, small boils, papular, pustular and corroding ulcers.

III. Suited to (Allen-153)

Large persons inclined to obesity, loss of sensibility, uncertain gait. Loss of memory; had to be told the word before he could speak it. Hands constantly busy; all sorts of fearful delusions; walks the room groaning, bemoaning his fate; full of fear, unsteady. Fits of uncontrollable weeping and profound melancholic delusions. Depressed; low spirited, Nervous anxiety. Night terrors of children (not from indigestion) with screaming.

IV. Clinical (Clarke-II-99)

Acne, Aphasia, Apoplexy, Asthma, Cholera infantum, Chordee, Colic, Diabetes, Emissions, Epilepsy, Erythema nodosum, General paralysis of insane, Haemorrhoids, Impotence, Laryngeal crises, Laryngismus, Locomotor ataxy, Nightmare, Nose-eruption on, Ovaries-affections of, Paralysis, Paralysis agitans, Polypi (rectal), Psoriasis, Screaming,

Sebaceous cysts, Seborrhoea, Self-abuse, Sensibility-loss of, Sleeplessness, Somnambulism, Speech-affections of, Syphilis, Tetanus, Urine-incontinence of.

V. **Symptoms-Particular** (Nash-456)

1. 'Fidgety hands'.
2. Sleeplessness is overcome by moving finger over bed cloth.
3. Plays with things to overcome nervousness.
   Zinc.-Fidgety Feet.
   Phos.-general fidgetiness or uneasiness.

VI. **Black Letter Symptoms** (Tyler-466-467)

- Loss of memory, had to be told before he could speak it.
- Hands constantly busy, all sorts of fearful delusions, walks groaning, bemoaning his fate, full of fear, unsteady.
- Fits of uncontrollable weeping and profound melancholia delusions.
- Depressed, low-spirited, nervous anxiety.
- Night terrors of children (not from indigestion) with screaming.
- Unconsciousness of what is happening around them. Cannot be recognized or be comforted by their friends. Sometimes followed by squinting.
- Seminal emissions, with depressed spirits, dull thought, bachache, staggering gait and great weakness.
- Nervous, restless, cannot sit still, but must move about, or otherwise occupy oneself; often suits nervous women.
- Spasm: from fright, anger, or other emotional causes, occuring in plethoric, nervous persons, or in women at the time of menses, during parturition, from sexual excitement. Too great reflex excitability. Sleeplessness, during teething, whooping-cough or laryngitis stridulus, from Bright's disease.
- Sleepless: restless, can only calm herself by incessant occupation.

- Night terrors of children, grina teeth in sleep, moans, cries, horrible dreams.
- Loss of sensibility-of body generally; of fauces, larynx, urethra, etc.

KALI CARBONICUM

I. Introduction (Cow-418)

Synonym: Potassium Carbonate.
Common Name: Carbonate of potash.
Preparation: Triturations.

It was first proved by Hahnemann in 30th potency. (Pierce-536).

II. General Analysis (Cow.)

Acts especially upon the respiratory mucous membranes, digestive tract, and with ovario-uterine systems. Causes excessive irritation bordering on inflammation. Chief expressions-sharp stitching pains, anaemia with dry skin and lack of perspiration (3-4 AM. Aggravation). Hair dry, fall out, Cures dandruff (Pierce-537).

III. Suited to (Allen-155)

Diseases of old people, dropsy and paralysis, with dark hair lax fibre, inclined to obesity (Amm. c., Graph.). After loss of fluids or vitality, particularly in anaemic (Cinchona rub., Phos. ac., Phos., Psor.) persons. Pains, stitching, darting, < rest, lying on affected side (Reverse of Bry.) Bag like swelling between upper eyelids and eyebrows (Apis.-lower).

IV. Clinical (Clarke-II-106)

Amenorrhoea, Anaemia, Asthma, Axilla-perspiration of, Backache, Biliousness, Bronchitis, Catarrh, Change of life, Chilblains, Clavus, Colds, Consumption, Cough, Debility, Dropsy, Dysmenorrhoea, Dyspepsia, Ear-inflammation of, Eyes-inflammation of; oedema around, Face-blotches on, Fear, Freckles, Gastralgia, Haemorrhage, Haemorrhoids, Hair-affections of, Headache, Heart affections, Hip-joint disease, Hydrothorax, Hysteria, Kidney-affections of, Knee-affections of; white swelling of, Larynx-catarrh of, Leucorrhoea, Liver-affections of, Lumbago, Menorrhagia, Metrorrhagia, Pleurisy, Pleurodynia, Pregnancy-affections of, Proctalgia, Sciatica, Sleeplessness, Spinal irritation, Stomach-affections of, Throat sore, Toothache, Typhoid, Urine-frequent passing of, Urticaria, Uterus-cancer of, Vertigo, Wens, Whooping-cough.

V. **Symptoms-General** (Nash-127)

1. Stitching pains, very characteristic.
2. Pains in lower right chest through to back.
3. Anaemia with bloating, especially upper eyelids, which hang down like a bag of water (lower-Apis.).
4. Backache, sweat, weakness very great: drops down in a chair.
5. Flatulence great; everything turns to gas.
6. Heart weak, irregular, intermits.
7. Modalities; < at 3 to 4 AM.
8. After loss of fluids or of vitality, particularly in the anaemic.
9. Asthma, relived when sitting up or bending forward, or by rocking (Ars.) worse from 2 to 4 AM.
10. Backache, before and during menses.
11. Complementary to Carb. v.

VI. **Symptoms-Particular** (Nash-127-131)

1. Pains-stitching, lower right chest, throat, asthma, pain runs to back, anaemia, 3 AM aggravation. Debility, nervous. *Key*-bags on upper eyelid. Puerperal fever, Phthisis Pulmonism with stitching pains-sudden and sharp.
2. Stitching Pains independent of movement, reverse of Bry.

   Kali c.-anywhere, any time, even to teeth, favourite is lower right chest.

   Bry.-on motion only, in serous membranes lying; is followed well by Kali c..
3. Pain in right lower chest-favourite locality

   Kali c.,

Merc. v.-sweat without relief, tongue and mouth.

4. Anaemia-(bags over upper eyelid, easy sweat, backache) of young girls, do not menstruate because of anaemia and general weakness. Bloating in face around eyes-upper lids with much pain in lumbar region (after Ferr. and Puls. when not indicated).
5. Debility-muscular. Menopause, old age, weak heart, constant backache-feels that back and legs must give out. Drops in a chair completely exhausted.
6. Fish Bone Sensation in throat (Hep. s., Dolichos., Nit. ac., Arg. n.).
7. Dyspeptic condition in broken down, aged people, anaemic.
   - Great sensitiveness of epigastric region externally.
   - Stomach distended, sensitive, as if it would burst.
   - Excessive flatulence, every thing he eats turns into gas.
   - Fullness, heat and great distension in the stomach, immediately after eating a little.
   - Stomach distended with wind after eating (Carb. v., China, Lyc.).
8. Worse lying on affected side.

   Bry. reverse of it.
9. Chief indicators:
   a) Bag-like swelling in the upper eyelids.
   b) Constant bachache-drops down in a chair.
   c) < 3 AM, 3-4 AM.
   d) Broken down, anaemic people, old persons.
   e) Weakened condition of muscles and nerves (easily frightened, cannot bear to be touched).
   f) Distended abdomen. Everything turns to gas.

VII. Black Letter Symptoms
(Tyler-472-474)

- Puffiness, swelling between eyebrows and lids, like a sac.
- Nose swollen, hard, red from tip to root.
- Swelling of face, especially over eyes. Stitches in middle of eye.

- Difficult swallowing: food descends oesophagus slowly and particles of food easily get into windpipe.
- Desire for sleep, during a meal.
- Dyspepsia of aged persons rather inclined to obesity, or after great loss of vitality; repugnance to all food; constant chilliness, cold hands and feet, no sweat however great the heat.
- Stitch pain in right abdomen, worse from motion.
- Cutting pain left upper abdomen, extending from lower left chest, where there is a sticking at the same time.
- Inflammation, soreness, stitches and tingling as from ascarides in varices of rectum.
- Anal fistula.
- Menses too early, scanty, of pungent odour, acrid, covering thighs with an itching eruption.
- Violent colicky pain in abdomen before menses, constipation during.
- Pressing and bearing down of pregnant females, as if a load were falling into the pelvis (Sep., Lil. t., etc.).
- Violent pain in the small of the back in pregnant females.
- Impending abortion with pains from back into buttocks and thighs; discharge of coagula; habitual; during the second or third month.
- Labour pains insufficient. Violent backache; wants back pressed (Sep.). Bearing down from back into pelvis.
- The pains are stitching and shooting, or they are in the back, shooting down into glutei muscles or pass on down thighs.
- Difficult wheezing breathing.
- Asthma: must lean forward with head on knees; worse in AM.
- Terrible attacks of asthma, worse at 3 AM.
- Cough at 3 AM., repeated every half-hour.
- Cutting pain in chest; in evening; after lying down; does not know how she shall lie; worse lying on right side; in AM. in lower part of chest especially in left side; moving into epigastrium and leaving a stinging sensation in left chest.

- Stitches in sides of chest on inspiration.
- Sticking pressure in left chest on breathing.
- Persons suffering from ulceration of lungs can scarcely get well without this anti-Psoric. (Hahnemann).
- Insufficiency-mitral valves.
- Tendency to fatty degeneration of heart.
- Sharp pains in small of back, with very acute labour-like pains running through to front at intervals of a few minutes, occasionally shooting down to glutei muscles.
- Backache while walking: feels must give up and lie down.
- Back: sharp stitching pains awaken him at 3 AM., he must get up and walk about; pains shoot from loins into nates.
- Stitching and shooting pains in back, shooting down into gluteal region or hips.
- Great tendency to start-starts with a loud cry.
- Cannot bear to be touched: starts when touched ever so lightly, especially on feet.
- Sensation of lump rolling over and over on coughing, rising from right abdomen to throat and back again.
- Liability to cold; inability to perspire; or great inclination to sweat; night sweats.
- Frequent exhaustion: feels she must lie down, or sit.
- Debility and desire to lie down.
- Wakes about I or 2 AM, cannot sleep again.
- Awaking about 2 AM and 4 PM with nearly all ailments, but especially those of throat and chest.
- Pains stitching, darting, worse during rest and lying on effected side. (The opposite to Bry., whose stitching pains are better from rest and from lying on affected side).
- Oppression of breathing accompanies most complaints.
- Anaemia with great debility, skin watery, milky-white.

KALI IODATUM

I. Introduction (Cow.-427)

Synonym: Kali Hydriodicum.
Common Name: Iodide of potash.
Preparation: A solution of 1 part to 99 of distilled water makes 2x dilution. Also Triturations.

It was first proved by Hartlaub and Trinks of Germany (Pierce-543).

II. General Analysis (Cow.)

Acts upon mucous tissues and glands, it resembles action of Mercury and involving disorganizing of fluids and destruction of tissues. It produces thickness of periosteum, hence useful in syphilitic nodes. Action on lymphatic and glandular systems resembles that of Iodine. It causes catarrhal inflammation with free secretion and little fever.

III. Clinical (Clarke-II-127)

Actinomycosis, Aneurism, Anidrosis, Bright's disease, Bubo, Bunions, Cancer, Caries, Colds, Condylomata, Consumption, Cough, Croup, Debility, Dropsy, Ears-otalgia; tinnitus, Emaciation, Erythema nodosum, Eyes-affections of; cysts on lids of, Fibroma, Glandular swellings, Gonorrhoea, Gout, Gumma, Haemorrhage, Hay-fever, Housemaid's knee, Influenza, Intra-menstrual haemorrhage, Joint affections, Laryngitis, Liver-diseases of, Locomotor ataxy, Lumbago, Lungs-hepatisation of; oedema of, Menstruation disordered, Neuralgia, Nodes, Noises in ears, Nystagmus, Odour of body-abnormal, Oedema glottidis, Pancreatitis, Paralysis, Pleurisy, Prostate-affections of, Rheumatism, Rickets, Rupia, Sciatica, Scrofula, Small-pox, Spine-Pott's curvature of, Spleen, Syphilis, Tic douloureux, Tongue-neuralgia of, Tumours, Ulcer, Wens.

IV. **Symptoms-General** (Nash-136)

1. Cough with profuse, thick, green, salty expectoration, from deep down, as if from mid-sternum, with pain through to back; great weakness and night sweats.
2. Stitches through the lungs; in middle of sternum; through sternum to back or deep in chest < walking.
3. Irresistible desire for open air; walking in open air does not fatigue; periosteal rheumatism.
4. Intolerable bone pain, especially at night; syphilitics.
5. Syphilitic affections, especially after the abuse of mercury.
6. Glandular swelling; interstital infiltration.
7. Hep. s. antidotes its over-use.

V. **Symptoms-Particular** (Nash-137)

1. Long continued cough after a hard cold or after an attack of pneumonia, as if patient running into consumption. Profuse expectoration from low down deep in the chest, with pain through to between the shoulders (Kali bich.). (Kali c.-lower right chest through back); exhausting night sweats and great general weakness. (Repeated cure by Nash of such cases where consumption seemed inevitable).
2. Sang. and Stan. have almost similar symptoms. In all three expectoration is profuse and thick.
   In Stan.-it tastes sweet.
   In Sang.-sputa and breath both foetid even to patient (Sep., Psor.).
   In Kali hydro. and Stan.-thick green, but in Sang.-not so much.
   In Kali hydro.-sometimes green, frothy, soap-suds like sputa.

KALI SULPHURICUM

I. Introduction (Cow-830.)

Synonym: Potassium Sulphate. Kali Sulphate.
Common Name: Sulphate of Potassium, Vitriolated water.
Preparation: Trituration.

II. General Analysis (Cow.)

Especially applicable to the later stages of inflammation, and to the ailments of acute desquamation (removal of outer layer of epidermis of the skin by scaling). Oxahiria.

III. Clinical (Clarke-II-159)

Antrum of Highmore-disease of, Asthma, Cataract, Catarrh, Chorea, Dandruff, Dyspepsia, Eczema, Epithelioma, Eustachian catarrh, Gleet, Gonorrhoea, Itch, Nails diseased, Nettlerash, Ozaena, Polypi, Psoriasis, Rheumatism, Rhus poisoning, Vertigo, Whooping-cough.

IV. Symptoms-General (Nash-374)

1. Yellow or greenish discharges from mucous membranes; cough loose and rattling.
2. Rheumatic pains in joints; moving from joint to joint.
3. Modalities-< in warm room; in the evening, > in open air.
4. The chronic of Puls.

V. Symptoms-Particular (Nash)

1. Evening aggravation of fever symptoms.
2. Kali s. = Puls., in Catarrh of mucous membranes when Puls. has failed.

KALMIA LATIFOLIA

I. Introduction (Cow-434)

Synonym: Kalmia Latifolia.
Natural Order: Ericaceae.
Common Name: Mountain Laurel.
Habitat: An evergreen shrub growing on rocky hills and damp soil from Maine to Ohio, Kentucky.
Preparation: Tincture from fresh leaves.

It was first proved by Hering (Pierce-549).

II. General Analysis (Cow.-436)

Acts prominently upon heart causing slow and weak pulse; upon nervous and muscular system, producing neuralgic and rheumatic pains, numbness, tingling and restlessness. Angina pectoris. Neuralgic pains attended with great weakness or numbness of the affected parts (Acon.).

III. Suited to (Allen-157)

Acute neuralgia, rheumatism, gouty complaints with heart involved, as a sequel of rheumatism or gout, pains sticking, darting, pressing, shooting, downwards (upwards-Cact., Led.). Numbness of the affected parts (Acon., Cham., Plat.).

IV. Clinical (Clarke-II-162)

Angina pectoris, Blindness, Bright's disease, Dropsy, Dysmenorrhoea, Gastralgia, Globus hystericus, Gout, Headache, Heart-disease of, Herpes zoster-neuralgia after, Keratitis, Leucorrhoea, Locomotor ataxy, Lumbago, Neuralgia, Paraplegia, Ptosis, Pregnancy-albuminuria of, Retinitis albuminurica, Rheumatism, Rumination, Scleroderma, Sclerotitis, Somnambulism, Sun-headaches, Syphilitic sore throat, Tinnitus, Tobacco-effect of, Vertigo, Vomiting.

V. **Symptoms-Particular** (Nash-227)

Has almost similar symptoms like Spig. so far as neuralgic symptoms are con-cerned. The sides and times of aggravation are different. Kalm. is often Right sided and Spig. left sided. Kalm. often does not involve whole head like Spig.

1. Neuralgic pains sometimes with numbness (esp. of face)-or followed by numbness.
   Kalm.-Right sided.
   Spig.-Left sided.

(For numbness-Kalm. is to be compared with Acon., Cham., Graph., Plat.).

2. Pain in Eyes esp., on turning them.
   Kalm.-has sense of stiffness (Rhus t., Nat. m.), Eyes hurt as if too big for the orbit.
   Spig.
3. Heart problem with slowness of pulse-Kalm., Dig., Spig., violent action of heart.
4. Rheumatism, migratory pains, with heart problem. Pains in Kalm. shift suddenly.
   Kalm.-From above downward (Cact.). Pain often extends down to the left hand (Rhus t.).
   Led.-From below upward.
   Puls.-For migratory rheumatism, with heart problem, Kalm. should come before Puls.

KREOSOTUM

I. Introduction (Cow-437)

Synonym: Creosotum.

Common Name: Wood Tor. Creosote, Kreosote.

Preparation: Dilution. One part of beech wood tar into 99 parts of Alcohol
= 2x dilution.

It was proved either by Dr. Syrbius of Germany or Dr. Whale of Italy. (Pierce-552).

II. General Analysis (Cow.)

Acts esp. upon lymphatic system and the mucous membranes of the digestive and female generative organs, and upon the skin, producing catarrhal conditions. Chief expression is corrosive, acrid, character of its secretions.

III. Suited to (Allen-157)

Dark complexioned, slight, lean, ill developed, poorly nourished, overgrown, very tall for her age (Phos.). Children looking old wrinkled (Abrot.) scrofulous or Psoric, rapid emaciation (Iod.), Haemorrhagic diathesis (Crotal. h., Lach., Phos.). Post climacteric diseases of women.

IV. Clinical (Clarke-II-176)

Acne, Amenorrhoea, Cancer, Carbuncles, Change of life, Cholera infantum, Coccygodynia, Congenital syphilis, Constipation, Consumption, Dentition, Diarrhoea, Ear affections , Enuresis, Epithelioma, Eructations, Eruptions, Flushing, Gastromalacia, Glossitis, Haemorrhage , Haemorrhagic diathesis, Herpes, Hysterical vomiting, Irritation, Leucorrhoea, Lip-epithelioma of, Lupus, Menstruation disordered, Neuralgia, Ovaries-affections of, Prostate-irritation of, Pregnancy-vomiting of, Pustules, Rheumatism, Sea-sickness, Stomach-affections of, Syphilis, Syphilitic deafness, Teeth carious, Toothache, Ulcer, Urine-incontinence of, Uterine affections, Vomiting, Whooping-cough, Yawning.

V. Symptoms-General (Nash-369)

1. Cholera Infantum; profuse vomiting; cadaverous smelling stools.
2. Haemorrhagic diathesis; small wound bleeds profusely (Phos.).
3. Acrid, foetid, decomposed, mucous secretions, sometimes ulcerating, bleeding, malignant.
4. Gums painful, dark red or blue; teeth decay as soon they come.
5. Sudden urge to urinate or during first sleep, which is very profound.

VI. Symptoms-Particular (Nash-370-372)

1. Bad teeth and painful, swelling, dark red or blue gums (better than Merc. c.)+.
2. Foetid corrosive discharge, leucorrhoea-yellow stain.
3. Great debility.
4. Obstinate haemorrhage-Haemorrhage occur with leucorrhagial trouble, intermittent, stop and come again and again. Lochia after confinement (Rhus t., Sul.,).
5. Cholera Infantum with dentition-incessant vomiting with cadaverous stool.
6. Tooth decays as soon as it comes, a mouthful of decayed teeth (esp. child) with spongy painful gums has best friend in Kreos.
7. Urine strong urge, esp. in sleep-wets bed while sleeping sound.

   Kreas.,

   Sep.
8. Urinary:-

   Can urinate only when lying, has copious pale urine.

   Can urinate-when sitting bent back-Zinc..

   Sudden urge-can't wait-Petrosel.

   Child wets bed during first sleep (very sound) can hardly

wake up (Sep.).

9. Menses of young girls.
10. Vomiting of pregnancy and intractable disease of stomach called gastromalacia. One of the best remedies.

VII. Black Letter Symptoms
(Tyler-478-480)

- Chronic swelling of eyelids and their margins; agglutination of lids.
- Lupus on NOSE: left side.
- Bad odour from decayed TEETH.
- Toothache; extending to temple and left face: drawing, extending to inner ear and temples: caused by caries.
- Teeth show dark specks and begin to decay as soon as they appear.
- Gums, bluish red, soft, spongy, easily bleeding, inflammed, ulcerated, scorbutic.
- Putrid odoar from MOUTH.
- VOMITING of sweetish water: undigested food; with dimness of vision: of large quantities of sour, acrid fluid, or white foamy mucous.
- Water, after it is swallowed, tastes bitter.
- Painful hard spot, at or to left of stomach.
- Frequent urging to URINATE, with copious, pale discharge; at night; can't get out of bed quick enough.
- Urinate six or seven times a day, always with great haste, and always passing a great deal.
- Smarting and burning in pudenda during and after micturition.
- LEUCORRHOEA of a yellow colour, also stains linen yellow, with great weakness of limbs.
- Leucorrhoea, if white, has odour of green corn.
- Burning between pudenda after urinating.
- Soreness between pudenda, with burning biting pains, as in little children.
- Violent itching of vagina, obliged to rub it. Posteriorly there is smarting: external genitalia swollen, hot and hard.
- On urinating, vagina pains as if sore; in the evening.
- Violent itching and biting between the Labia: she

could not refrain from rubbing.

- Corrosive itching between pudenda and in vagina: so that she was obliged to rub them; with a feeling of burning and swelling in the pudenda.
- Scirrhus of vagina, painful to touch.
- Inveterate ulcers on neck of uterus.
- Severe headache before and during menses.
- Her hoemorrhage seems to pass into a corrosive, ichorus discharge and then to freshen up again and go on.
- During pregnancy, nausea and vomiting; ptyalism, vomiting of sweet water.
- Lochia: blackish, lumpy, very offensive; excoriating; almost ceasing, freshens up again; persistent, brown and offensive.
- Left THUMB pains as if sprained and stiff.
- SKIN: itching; towards evening so violent as to drive one almost wild.

LAC CANINUM

I. Introduction (Allen)

Common Name: Bitch's Milk.

II. Suited to (Allen-162)

Nervous, restless, highly sensitive organism, symptoms erratic, pains constantly flying from one part to another (Kali bich., Puls.), changing from side to side every few hours or days very forgetful, absent minded (Agn. cast., Anac., Caust., Nat. m.).

III. Clinical (Clarke-II-189)

Arms-varicosis of, Breasts painful, Chancre, Croup, Diphtheria, Dysmenorrhoea, Epulis, Eye affections, Gonorrhoea, Headache, Ichthyosis, Leucorrhoea, Neuralgia, Ovaries-affections of, Ranula, Rheumatism, Sciatica, Spinal irritation, Stomach-affections of, Syphilis, Throat sore, Ulcer, Uterine affections, Vaccinosis, Veins-varicose , Warts.

IV. Symptoms-General (Nash-372)

1. Inflammatory affections travel crosswise, from side to side, back and forth (rheumatism, sore throat etc.).
2. Breasts and throat get sore at every menstrual period.
3. Mastitis; breasts very sore and tender; can't bear a jar of the bed; on stepping has to hold them up, on going down stairs.

V. Symptoms-Particular (Nash-372)

1. Pain alternates side to side, back to forth also crosswise (when Puls. fails).

2. Sore throat alternates with pain in the limbs (when Rhus t. fails).
3. Menses gushes instead of continuous flow with sore throat and breast.
4. Breasts sore to least jar, has to hold them in hand (Mastitis).
5. Sensation of urination during sleep-urine would escape if bladder was not strong enough (Clarke-Dictionary of Materia Medica).

VI. Black Letter Symptoms
(Tyler-490-491)

- Swallowing very difficult, painful, almost impossible.
- Soreness of throat begins with a tickling sensation, which causes constant cough; then sensation of lump on one side, causing constant deglutition; this condition entirely ceases only to commence on the opposite side and often alternates again returning to its first condition; these sore throats are very apt to begin and end with the menses.
- Tonsils inflamed and very sore, red and shining, almost closing throat; dryness of fauces and throat; swelling of sub-maxillary glands.
- Diptheritic membrane white like china; mucous membrane of throat glistening as if varnished; membranes leave one side and to the other repeatedly, Desire for warm drinks which may return through the nose. Post diptheritic paralysis.
- Serviceable in almost all cases where it is required to dry up milk.
- When walking seems to be walking on air; when lying does not seem to touch the bed.
- Erratic disposition of symptoms; pains constantly flying from one part to another.

Other notable symptoms

- Great fear: of failing downstairs: of inability to perform duties. Fear of death, with anxious face.
- Wakes distressed; must rise and occupy herself. Fear she will be crazy: that any symptom is some settled

disease; that everything she says is a lie: that she is looked down by everyone: that she is of no importance: that she is dirty: that she ears someone else's nose: that she sees spiders.

- That she is surrounded by myriads of snakes, some running like lightning up and down inside skin; some inside feel long and thin. Fears to step on floor lest she should tread on them, and make them squire and wind round her legs (Arg. n., Sep.). Fears to look behind her lest she should see snakes: is seldom troubled with them after dark.
- On going to bed, afraid to shut her eyes lest a large snake should hit her in the face (Bell.). Has most horrid sights presented to her mental vision (not always snakes). Horribly afraid they will show themselves to her natural eye. Fear lest pimples would prove little snakes, and twine and twist round each other.
- Feels that she is a loathsome, horrible mass of disease: could not near to look at any part of her body. Even hands as it intensified the feeling of disgust and horror.
- Could not bear any part of her body to touch another, could not bear one finger to touch another. If she could not get out of her body, she would soon become crazy.
- Feels that heart or breathing would stop; frightens herself, which makes heart palpitate. Fancies he is going out of the mind.
- Looks under chairs, table, sofa, expecting some horrible monster to creep forth; feels that it would drive her mad. Not afraid in the dark; only imagines she sees them in the light.
- Feels that she is going to become unconscious: wakes with sensation of bed in motion.
- Dreamed of a large snake in her bed (Bell.).
- Dreams often that she is urinating: Wakes to find herself on the point of doing so (Sep). s

LACHESIS

I. Introduction (Cow-440)

Synonym: Lachesis Mutus.
Natural Order: Ophidia
Common Name: Bush master snake of Brazil.
Preparation: Triturations of the venom.

Herring collected the venom in Brazil in 1828 and case records were published in 1835 and 1837 (Pierce-557).

II. General Analysis (Cow.)

Acts upon cerebro-spinal system and more upon Pneumogastric, system. The nerve centres are poisoned, causing prostration, Convulsion, and unconsciousness ensue. From pneumogastric-irritable throat, larynx bronchi and heart and yet not into distinct inflammations, abscess, gangrene, pyaemia and general typhoid conditions. Chief expression-aggravation of all symptoms after sleep.

III. Suited to (Allen-159)

Melancholy temperament, dark eyes, low spirits and indolence. Women-choleric temperament with freckles and red hair (Phos.) Emaciated than fleshy; those changed mentally and physically by their illness. Climacteric-hot flushes, hot perspiration, burning headache. Ailments-from a long lasting grief, fright, disappointed love (Aur. m., Ign., Phos. ac.) Headache-bursting < motion, pressure, stooping, weight on vertex (Sep.). Anything coming close to nose or mouth interferes with breathing. Fanned slowly (Carb. v.-fast). As soon as falls sleep-breathing stops (Amm. c., Grind., Lac can., Op.). Trembling-from weakness-moving (Sul., Tuberc.). Small wounds bleed freely (Crotal. h., Kreas., Phos.), Boils, Bladder-a ball rolling in as if, Fever returns each year-each spring (Carb. v., Sul.) Left sided medicine.

IV. Clinical (Clarke-II-210)

Albuminuria, Alcoholism, Amblyopia, Aneurism, Apoplexy, Appendicitis, Asthenopia, Asthma, Atheroma, Bed-sores, Boils, Bubo, Caecum-inflammation of, Carbuncles, Catalepsy, Chancre, Change of life, Chilblains, Ciliary neuralgia, Cough, Cyanosis, Delirium tremens, Diphtheria, Dog-bite, Dropsy, Dyspepsia, Ears-polypi of; wax in; noises in, Enteric fever, Epilepsy, Erysipelas, Eyes-affections of; haemorrhage into, Fainting, Fistula lachrymalis, Flatulence, Fungus haematoides, Gall-stones, Gangrene, Glanders, Gum-bleeding of, Haemorrhage, Haemorrhoids, Hay-fever, Headache, Heart affections, Heartburn, Hemiplegia, Hernia, Herpes facialis, Hoarseness, Hydrophobia, Hysteria, Injuries, Intermittent fever, Jaundice, Labour-pains after, Laryngismus, Laryngitis, Leprosy, Liver-affections of, Locomotor ataxy, Malignant pustule, Measles, Meniere's disease, Mercury-effects of, Mind-affections of, Morvan's disease, Mouth sore, Mumps, Neuralgia, Neurasthenia, Nymphomania, Oedema of lungs, Otorrhoea, Ovaries-affections of, Paralysis, Paraphimosis, Perityphlitis, Perspiration-bloody; absent, Phlegmasia alba dolens, Plague, Pneumonia, Puerperal fever and convulsions, Purpura, Pyaemia, Quinsy, Rabies, Scarlatina, Sciatica, Scurvy, Small-pox, Stings, Strangury, Syphilis, Throat sore, Trachea-affections of, Traumatic fever, Tumours, Ulcer, Veins-varicose, Vertigo, Vicarious menstruation (nose bleed), Warts, Whitlow, Wounds.

V. Symptoms-General (Nash-111)

1. Feels very sad and despondent: < after sleeping, or in the morning.
2. Enemy of all constriction; must loosen everything (neck, chest, throat, abdomen, etc.).
3. Left-sided affections generally, especially throat, chest ovaries.
4. Inflamed parts very tender to touch and of bluish or dark colour.
5. Great weakness and trembling; tongue trembles, when protruding it; catches under the teeth (lower).

6. Blood decomposes, breaks down, Haemorrhage; blood uncoagulable; ulcers and even slight wounds bleed profusely.
7. Modalities; < at climacteric; touch constriction or pressure, sun-heat, after sleeping; > after discharges (suppressed or delayed discharges).
8. Many complaints connected with the menopause; hot flushes, hot sweats, burning vertex headaches, haemorrhoids, Haemorrhage.
9. Great physical and mental exhaustion; trembling in whole body, would constantly sink from weakness.

VI. Symptoms-Particular (Nash-112-124)

1. After sleep worse.
2. Enemy of all constrictions.
3. Left sides-esp. throat, chest, ovaries.
4. Alternates excitation and depression (alternate action on mind and sensorium) Loquacity, rapid change of subjects.
5. Chronic mania, fever, weak memory, confusions to time (depression).
6. Sun-Headache with pale face, sleeps into headache.
   Lach.-follows Glon. well, every time when goes out in sun.
   (one of the best remedies).
   Glon.-Immediate effects of sun stroke.
   Nat. c.-chronic headache when ever exposed to sun. (Nat. m.).

(a) Pressure on vertex (esp. at Menopause).
   Lach.-burning on the vertex (Sul.). Headache extending into nose,
   mostly in acute catarrh, when the discharge is suppressed or
   stops after sleep.
      Cact.,
      Glon.,
      Menyanthes.

(b) Sleeps into headache. Dreads sleep, as awakens with distressing headache.

(c) Headache extending to nose, when coryza stopped, after sleep-often found in Hay-fever with frequent sneezing.

7. Alimentary Tract.

(a) Gum swollen, spongy. Easily bleeding (Merc. c.).

(b) Tongue very dry, trembles when protruded, catches under lower teeth.

Lach., Gels. (puts out with difficulty in the beginning of fever; in Lach. later) Gels.-not so dry as in Lach.

(c) Throat and neck sensitive to slightest touch (Sep.), even weight of bed covers, distresses about the throat.

Lach.,

Sep.,

-Empty or liquid or saliva swallowing is worse.

-Swallowing of solids does not aggravate so much.

-Pain runs into ears.

Lach. < hot drink in tonsilitis and diphtheria, swelling begins on left side.

Saba. > hot drink L-R on left side then extends to right (Sabad)

ENEMY OF ALL CONSTRICTIONS ANY WHERE IN BODY.

Lach. < pressure.

Bry. > pressure.

8. Throat-centre of this remedy.

9. Skin-Purple or bluish-best medicine.

10. Stool and Anus.

Lach.-As if anus closed, when he attempts, it so hurts, that gives up.

pressing for stool-offensive.

Nux. v.-like ineffectual urge.

Lyc.-like painful constriction.

11. Haemorrhoids of decomposed bloodduring acute, in exhausting disease like Typhoid. Throbbing-little hammer's beating in rectum (Haemorrhoids).

12. Female generative organs-left ovary (Neuralgia).

Lyc.-Right ovary.

13. Uterine trouble-Pain increases till relieved by bleeding from vagina-then again after few hours or days

and same again L to R (Reverse-Lyc.) Intolerance of least contact over region, womb proplases, hot flashes, pale face.

Crotal. h.,–post climacteric problem- hot flashes, hot vertex, pale, fainlug.

Lach., *best remedies.* Bleeding tem-face, fainting, deranged.

Kreosot. *porarily relieves* sufferings. capillary circulation esp.

Haemorrhage.

14. Cough.

-Dry hacking cough < touch < during sleep. (when -Cham. fails).

-Cough with pain in Anus or stitch in piles.

-Short dry cough with heart problem, constriction sensation being the

guiding symptom.

15. Nervous system.

-Trembling from extreme weakness, both mental and physical, < sleep or rest.

Lach.-with prostration
Gels.-weakness in early
} Paralysis of left side, as a result of stage apoplexy or cerebral exhaustion.

16. Sun, Heat-bad effects of, or worse from hot weather.

Lach.-Nervous system affected most profoundly.

Gels.-resembles

Lach.-Trembling morning. Prostration left sided paralysis.

Epilepsy. Locomotor ataxy.

Ant. c..,

Gels.,

Glon.,

Nat. c.,

Nat. m..

17. Sleeps into aggravation (any problem) shortness of breath. As soon as sleeps, breathing stops. Anything close to mouth stops breathing. Shortness of breath when walking.

Grind.,

Dig.

18. Tissues-swelling on all parts of body.
 (a) Bluish-going to black.
  Lach.,
  Tarent. cub.,
  Anthrac.
 (b) wound bleeds profusely, swollen, blood in urine in many conditions.
  Lach.-Left sided.
  Lyc.-Right sided.
19. Blood decomposes-often in Typhoid-Lach.
20. Skin affection attended with dark bluish characteristic colour.

VII. Black Letter Symptoms (Tyler-498-499)

- Loquacity.
- Vertigo on waking. Vertigo on closing the eyes.
- Headache extending to nose or to root of nose.
- Tearing, zygoma into ear.
- Hawking of mucous, with rawness of throat, after a nap in the daytime.
- Dry throat, in night, on waking.
- Pains in throat in connection with ears.
- Throat and larynx painful, even bending head backwards.
- Throat seems swollen as if two lumps as fists came together; on empty swallowing not on eating which seems to do good.
- Sensation of a crumb of bread in throat.
- Such a sore and ulcerated throat that she could with difficulty swallow.
- Sensitive throat, as if sore, with pain on left side.
- Liquids can be more easily swallowed than solids.
- Can endure nothing tight on the throat.
- Throat very sensitive to external pressure.
- Everything about the throat is distressing.
- If in the evening on lying down anything touches the throat or larynx, it seems as if he would suffocate and the pain is worse.

- Throat sensitive, even to the touch of the linen.
- Larynx painful to touch: whole throat painful to touch.
- A feeling as if something were swollen in pit of throat and would suffocate him: it can't be swallowed: with soreness of throat.
- Cough worse after every sleep.
- Cough caused by pressure on larynx.
- Dry, hacking cough, caused by touching the throat: also occurring after sleep at night.
- Constantly obliged to take a deep breath.
- During heat, as of orgasm of blood, obliged to loosen the clothes about the neck, as though they hindered the circulation of the blood, with a suffocative feeling.
- Beating in the anus as with little hammers.
- Diarrhoea followed by throbbing as with little hammers in the anus.
- Cramp-like pain in precordial region, causing palpitation and anxiety.
- Weakness of whole body, on rising in the morning.
- Great physical and mental exhaustion.
- Obliged to open the clothes, which affords relief (with faintness).
- Obliged to wear the clothes very loose, especially about the stomach; even in bed is obliged to loosen and raise the night dress in order to avoid pressure; she dares not even lay arm across the body on account of the pressure.

LEDUM PALUSTRE

I. Introduction (Cow 457)

Synonym: Ledum Palustre.
Natural Order: Ericaceae.
Common Name: Marsh Tea, Wild Rosemary.
Habitat: An ever growing shrub in moist swampy grounds in Europe and Asia etc.
Preparation: Tincture from the fresh herb.

It was proved first by Hahnemann (Pierce-565).

II. General Analysis (Cow.)

Acts upon serous, fibrous and mucous tissues; upon periostium; upon skin, producing inflammatory symptoms of rheumatic or arthritic character, causing a deposit of solid, earthy masses in the tissues. A valuable remedy in rheumatic and arthritic affections (Cow.-549).

III. Suited to (Allen-167)

Rheumatic, gouty diathesis (Bry.) constitutions abused by alcohol (Colch.), affects left shoulder and right hip joint (Agar., Ant. tar., Stram.). Rheumatic pains are < by motion < at night, by warmth of bed and covering; > only when feet in icy water (Sec.).

IV. Clinical (Clarke-II-262)

Ascites, Asthma, Bites, Black-eye, Bruises, Deafness, Ear-inflammation of, Eczema, Erythema nodosum, Face-pimples on, Feet-pains in; tender, Gout, Haemoptysis, Hands-pains in, Intoxication, Joints-affections of; Joints-cracking in, Meniere's disease, Pediculosis, Priapism, Prickly heat, Punctured wounds, Rheumatism, Skin-eruptions on, Stings, Tetanus, Tinnitus, Tuberculosis, Varicella, Whitlow, Wounds.

V. Symptoms-General (Nash-364)

1. Rheumatism begins in feet and travels upward (Kalm. opposite).
2. The swellings are pale, sometimes oedematous and < at night, in the heat of the bed; uncovering or cold water relives.
3. Ecchymosis; 'black eye' from a blow or contusion: better than Arn.
4. Rheumatism and rheumatic gout; joints become the seat of nodosities and 'gout stones' which are painful.
5. Complaints of people who are cold all the time; lack of animal or vital heat; parts cool to touch, but not cold subjectively to patient.
6. Punctured wounds by sharp-pointed instruments, rat bites, stings of insects, especially mosquitoes.

VI. Symptoms-Particular (Nash-365-368)

1. Rheumatism often begins in the back, extremities or joints and driven to heart, if not cured.
2. Rheumatism-cold goes upwards from feet.

   Led.-goes upward, Pale swelling < night, heat of bed (Merc. c.).

   Kalm.-goes downward < night.
3. Painful and sensitive soles, can hardly step on them.

   Ant. c.
Led.
Lyc.
Sil.
   } Ankles swollen, soles painful, sensitive.
Led. is unnaturally cold.
(Sil. but < not warmth of bed).
4. Injury-Pain in Eye ball (Symp.).

   Arn.-Led. sometimes finishes the work begun by Arn.

   Led.-Best remedy to remove black and blue spots of the blows received (Sul. ac.).

   Nux. v.-ecchymosis, turning into conjunctivitis (inner eyelid) specific medicine.
5. Punctured wounds-good remedy for.

   Led.-from a nail, sting, of insects, rat bite etc.

Hyper.-better if a nerve is wounded.
Rut.-if Periosteum is wounded.
Calc. phos. } to promote re-union.
Symp. } or repair of bones.

VII. Black Letter Symptoms
(Tyler 505-507)

- All day long, discontented with his fellow creatures, which at last amounted to misanthropy.
- Vertigo. Head tends to sink backwards.
- Considerable dilatation of pupils.
- Contusions or wounds of eye/lids especially with extravasation of blood.
- A noise in the ears like ringing of bells, or like a storm of wind, roaring in the ears, as from wind.
- Hard pressure inwards in the lower jaw.
- Sore throat, with fine shooting pain.
- A sudden flow of watery saliva from mouth with colic, water brash.
- Tight, painful respiration.
- Dyspnoeic constriction of chest, worse movement and walking.
- Chronic cough characterized by cold and deficiency of animal heat.
- Expectoration of bright red blood with violent cough.
- Pain in loins after sitting.
- On raising arm, extremely painful shooting in shoulder.
- Pressure in left shoulder joint, aggravated by movement.
- Trembling of the hands when grasping or when moving them.
- Whitlow, from punctured wounds, needle pricks, splinters.
- Pressure in left thigh, posteriorly; as if the muscles were not in their right places, like pain of dislocation; in every position, but especially violent when touched and when walking.
- Trembling of knees (and hands) when sitting and walking.

- Weakness in knee joints, when walking, a tearing pressure in them. Tearing pressure in right knee joint and below it; worse by walking.
- Swelling, and tensive and shooting pain in knees when walking.
- Pressure above left ankle, worse by movement.
- Very severe gnawing itching on dorsum of both feet; more violent after scratching; only allayed when he had scratched the feet raw: much aggravated by heat of bed.
- Obstinate swelling of the feet.
- Pressure on the inner ball of left foot.
- Soles of feet painful when walking as if filled with blood.
- Ball of big toes is soft swollen and painful when treading: tendons stiff.
- Gout, worse in feet: gouty nodosities on joints: fine tearing in toes.
- Pain in ankles as from strain or false step.
- Rheumatic pains going from below upwards: joints pale, swollen tense, hot; stinging, drawing pains. Worse from warmth of bed and bed covering; worse motion and in evening.
- Rheumatism and rheumatic gout; begins in lower limbs and ascends; especially if brought into a low, asthenic state by abuse of Colch. , joints become the seat of nodosites and "gout stones" which are painful.
- Swelling of feet and legs up to knees, purple and mottled, pitting on pressure with rending pains in periosteum; comfortable only when holding feet in ice water.
- Affects principally left shoulder and right hip joint.
- Rheumatism begins in lower limbs and ascends.
- Heat in the hands and the feet in the evening.
- Long continued warm sweat on hands and feet.
- Can't bear the heat of the bed, on account of heat and burning in the limbs.
- Gone to sleep feeling of the limbs.

- Uneasy dreams; he is sometimes in one place, sometimes in another, sometimes occupied with one subject, sometimes with another.
- Sleeplessness with restlessness and tossing about.
- On waking, slight sweat with itching all over that compelled scratching.
- Chilliness without subsequent heat: limbs extremely cold, while rest of body was warm.
- Rigor over whole back with rather hot cheeks and hot forehead, without redness of face or thirst; with cold hands.
- Sprains of ankles and feet.
- Punctured wounds, from sharp pointed instruments, as awls, rat bites nails, etc., particularly if wounded parts feel cold to touch and to patient.
- Punctured wounds; stings, of insects especially of mosquitoes.
- Rheumatic, gouty diathesis; constitutions abused by alcohol.
- Emaciation of suffering parts (Plumb.).

LILIUM TIGRINUM

I. Introduction (Cow-461)

Natural Order: Liliaceae.
Common Name: Tiger Lily.
Habitat: A garden plant of China, Japan.
Preparation: Tincture from the fresh plant.

It was first proved by Dr. W.E. Payne in1867 for homeopathy (Pierce-567).

II. Genral Analysis (Cow.)

Acts profoundly upon female generative organs and heart. In the former, produces irritation congestion and sub acute inflammation. In heart-depressed action of heart, cardiac irritation and palpitation. Chief expression is bearing down sensation in uterine region as if every thing would press out of the vagina.

III. Suited to (Allen-168)

Principally left-sided medicine. Tormented about her salvation (Lyc., Sul., Verat.) with ovarian/uterus complaints. Consolation < can hardly avoid weeping. Timid, fearful anxious about disease. Disposed to curse, to think obscene things (Anac., Lac can.) Listless yet can't sit still restless yet does not want to walk. Must keep busy to suppress sexual desire. Pain in small spot constantly shifting (Kali bich.). Bearing down sensation in abdomen and pelvic region (Lac can., Mur. p., Sep.).

IV. Clinical (Clarke-II-276)

Angina pectoris, Asthenopia, Astigmatism, Dementia, Diarrhoea, Dysentery, Eye affections, Fibroma, Heart-affections of; palpitation of, Hysteria, Ovaries-affection of; dropsy of, Pruritus vulvae, Spinal irritation, Urine-frequent passing of, Uterus-affections of; displacements of; subinvolution of.

V. Symptoms-General (Nash-207)

1. Great bearing down as if pelvic contents would press out through vagina; > by pressing up with the hand or sitting down (Sep. crosses the legs).
2. Sensation of constriction in heart with uterine troubles. Frequent desire for stool and urine with uterine displacements, tenesmus.
3. Tormented about her salvation.
4. Listless, yet does not want to sit still; restless, yet does not want to walk; hurried manner, desire to do something, yet no ambition; imperative duties, inability to perform them.
5. Depression of spirits; disposition to weep; aversion to food, indifferent about anything being done for her.

VI. Symptoms-Particular (Nash-208)

1. ***Lil. t.= Sep.*** (bearing down sensation common to both).

    Lil. t.-as if whole abdomen would come through vagina.

    Sep.-as if it would come down through uterine.
1. No remedy is more efficacious than Lil. t. in uterine displacement.
2. In Lil. t. there is more urinary irritation sometimes with rectal irritation (Merc. c., Caps., Nux. v.) frequent desire to urinate sometimes so severe that Canth. is reminded.
3. Heart held by Iron hand, as if
4. Sensation as if the heart were held by iron hand-Lil. t., Cact..
5. Tearfulness, Doubts her salvation

    Puls.,
    Lil. t.,
    Verat.,
    Sul.,
    Lyc.

6. Hurried feeling as of imperative duties with her inability to perform them.
   Lil. t.,
   Arg. n..

VII. Black Letter Symptoms (Tyler-512)

- Tormented about her salvation. Uterine complaints.
- Depression of spirits; profound; can hardly keep from crying.
- Disposition to weep, with nausea and pain in back; averse to food; weeps much and is very timid; indifferent about anything being done for her.
- Dragging down of whole Abdominal contents extending even to organs of chest; must support abdomen; as if whole contents were pushing down into a funnel; is compelled to cross her legs for fear everything would be pressed out.
- Bearing down sensation in pelvis as through everything was coming into world through vagina.
- Pressure in rectum, with almost constant desire to go to stool.
- Continuous pressure in region of Bladder, constant desire to urinate with scanty discharge, smarting in urethra and tenesmus.
- Frequent urination through day; with dull headache moving from sinciput to occiput, finally settling in left temple.
- If desire is not attended to, feeling of congestion of chest.
- Sharp pain in ovarian region; burning, stinging, cutting, grasping pain extends across hypogastrium to groin, down leg; bearing down when standing; sensitive to pressure; ovary swollen to nearly the size of a child's head.
- Severe neuralgic pain in Uterus, could not bear touch not even weight of bedclothes or slightest jar; anteversion.
- Anteversion and retrogression of uterus; patients nearly all have constipation.

- Sensation as if Heart was grasped or squeezed in a vice; as if blood had all gone to heart, producing a feeling as if he must bend double inability to walk straight.

LOBELIA INFLATA

I. Introduction (Cow-466)

Natural Order: Lobeliaceae.
Common Name: Indian Tobacco, Puke Root.
Habitat: Annual plant growing near road sides etc. and in neglected fields.
Preparation: Tincture from the fresh plant.

It was first proved for homeopathy by Dr. Jeanes of the USA. (Pierce-569).

II. General Analysis (Cow.)

Acts upon cerebrospinal system especially the pneumogastric nerves, producing prostration, oppression of the chest, nausea and vomiting. Spasm of larynx and bronchi, especially when with nausea.

III. Suited to (Allen-170)

Persons of light hair, blue eyes fair complexion, inclined to be fleshy. Gastric derangements-extreme nausea and vomiting, morning sickness; Headache afternoon to midnight. Sacrum-extreme sensitiveness, can't bear slightest touch, even of a soft pillow.

IV. Clinical (Clarke-II-302)

Alcoholism, Alopecia, Amenorrhoea, Angina pectoris, Asthma, Asthma Milleri, Cardialgia, Cough, Croup, Deafness, Debility, Diarrhoea, Dysmenorrhoea, Dyspepsia, Emphysema, Faintness, Gall-stones, Gastralgia, Haemorrhoidal discharge, Hay-asthma, Heart affections, Hysteria, Meningeal headaches, Morning sickness-of drunkards; of pregnancy, Morphia habit, Palpitation, Pleurisy, Psoriasis, Rigid os, Seborrhoea, Shoulder-pains in, Tea-effects of, Urethra-stricture of, Vagina-serous discharge from, Vomiting of pregnancy, Wens, Whooping-cough.

V. Symptom–Particular—Nausea
(Nash-471)

Vomiting with great relaxation of muscular system and profuse accumulation of saliva.

LYCOPODIUM CLAVATUM

I. Introduction (Cow.-468)

Synonym: Lycopodium.
Natural Order: Lycopodiaceae.
Common Name: Wolf's foot. Club Moss.
Habitat: A moss growing in all parts of the world, esp. in Northern countries.
Preparation: Trituration of the pollen of the plant.

It was first proved by Hahnemann (Pierce-570).

II. General Analysis (Cow.)

Acts powerfully upon vegetative system, causing a slowly advancing weakness of functional power of the tissue; upon mucous membranes of the respiratory, digestive, genito-urinary and upon skin, local action upon liver and digestive tract wherein causing disturbed digestion, hepatisation, constipation and upon kidneys uric acid diathesis, skin sluggish and unhealthy. Chief expression is excessive accumulation of flatus in the abdomen.

III. Suited to (Allen-171)

Intellectually keen, but physically weak, upper part of body emaciated lower semi-dropsical; Predisposed to lung and hepatic affections (Calc. c., Phos., Sul.) Deep seated chronic, progressive disease. Child—well developed hard with sickly body. Baby cries all day sleeps all night (Reverse of Jal., Psor.). Easily angered, miserable, malicious, irritable, on waking, cries when thanked (Puls.). Diphtheria-< after sleep and from cold drink (Warm drinks-Lach.). Dryness of vagina-burning during and after coition (Lyss.). Stool-discharge of blood with every stool. Hernia-R-sided best. Pneumonia-right lung. Waking at night feeling hungry (Cina., Psor.). < 4-8 PM. Right-sided medicine.

IV. Clinical (Clarke-II-329)

Abdomen distended, Abortion, Albuminuria, Aneurism, Angina pectoris, Aphasia, Asthma, Axilla-offensive perspiration of, Biliousness, Borborygmi, Bright's disease, Cancer, Cataract, Constipation, Consumption, Corns, Cough, Cramps, Cystitis, Debility, Diphtheria, Distension, Dropsy, Dysentery, Dysmenorrhoea, Dyspepsia, Ear-eczema of, Eczema, Ephelis, Epistaxis, Epithelioma, Excoriations, Eye-inflammation of; polypi of canthus, Face-eruption on, Feet perspiring, Fibroma, Flatulence, Gall-stone colic, Glands swollen, Goitre, Gout, Gravel, Haematuria, Haemorrhoids, Hair falling off, Hands chapped, Heartburn, Heart disease, Hemiopia, Hernia, Hydropericardium, Hypochondriasis, Hysteria, Impotence, Influenza, Intermittents, Intertrigo, Irritation, Labour pains abnormal, Lip-cancer of, Liver disorder, Liver-spots, Locomotor ataxy, Lung affections, Menstruation disordered, Metrorrhagia, Naevus, Nymphomania, Otorrhoea, Panaritium, Paralysis, Paralysis agitans, Peritonitis, Phlegmasia albs dolens, Physometra, Plica polonica, Pneumonia, Polypi-of eye; of ear; of nose, Proctalgia, Prostatitis, Pylorus-affections of, Quinsy, Renal colic, Rheumatism, Rhagades, Sciatica, Sleep abnormal, Speech-disordered, Stammering, Strains, Sunstroke, Taste abnormal, Throat sore, Tongue-coated; cramp in, Typhoid fever, Urine abnormal, Varicosis, Warts, Water-brash, Whooping-cough, Worms, Yawning.

V. Symptoms-General (Nash-57)

1. Depression of mind and sensorium, stupid; lower jaw drops; chronic conditions, memory fails; uses wrong words to express himself; messes up things; failing brain power.
2. Right sided complaints or begins on right and travels leftward; throat, ovaries, uterine region, kidney and skin troubles, hernia.
3. Sense of satiety or hunger, but soon fills up.
4. Great flatulence with rumbling, mostly intestinal and pressing downward.
5. Lithic acid diathesis, red sand in clear urine; > pains in back or kidneys after passing.

6. Dark complexioned people; emaciated in face and upper parts, bloated or swollen in lower. Keen intellectual, but feeble muscular development.
7. Modalities: < 4 to 8 PM after eating, in warm room > in cool open air, on motion.
8. Irritable, peevish and cross on waking; ugly; kick and scream easily angered; cannot endure opposition or contradiction seeks disputes; is beside himself.
9. One foot hot and the other cold.
10. Great thirst after the sweat.
11. Chill on left side of body (Caust., Carb. v.).
12. Sour vomiting between chill and heat, must uncover (Lach.).
13. Perspiration immediately after the chill; thirst after sweating stage.
14. In intermittents, flatulence; sour eructation. Sour taste, sour sweat, sour vomiting.
15. Complexion pale, dirty, unhealthy, sallow, looks older than he is.

VI. Symptoms-Particular (Nash-58-64)

1. Anti Psoric leading Trio of Hahnemann.

   Sul., Calc. c., Lyc.

   Lyc.—sallow, sunken, persons with premature line of age in face, looks older than he is. Children—sickly bodies, well developed heads, but puny, sickly bodies. Awake out of sleep ugly.
2. Flatulant Trio-Bloating in abdomen

   China—whole abdomen, constant fermentation going on in abdomen, loud croaking and rumbling.

   Lyc.—lower abdomen with fermentation flatulence with liver problem.

   Carb. v.—upper abdomen with left hypochondria or in region of colon.
3. Hunger with satiety, alternates—very characteristic of Lyc.

   A few mouthfuls fill him right up-Lyc.+++
4. Constipation.

   Nux. v.—irregular peristaltic (Contraction).

Lyc. —Spasmodic contraction of anus which prevents stool and causes pain.

5. Right sided hernia cured without truss.+++
6. Liver Troubles.

   Lyc.—Atrophy (reduced functioning).

   China-Hypertrophy (increase in size).
7. Urinary—Sand (red) in urine-calculi-Lyc. +++ after severe crying spell in adults, pain in back region of kidney > after discharge of sandy urine.

   Sarsa.,

   Sanic.,

   Bor.—child cries before urination.
8. Impotence.

   Lyc.—Strong desire but can't perform.

   Agn. cast.,

   Sel.,

   Calad.
9. Right sided remedy; most complaints travel Right to Left.

   Lach.
Lyc.
Lac can.
Phyt. } swelling, suppuration of tonsils, in old Quinsy subjects.

   (a) Diphtheria.

   Lyc.,

   Merc. proto.—also R to L with peculiar symptom.

   Brom.—begins below and goes up.

   Lyc.—begins up and travels down wards.
10. Nose block—breathes through mouth during night.

    Lyc.—Chronic dry catarrah of nose, completely closed, breathes through mouth.

    Amm. c.,

    Hep. s.,

    Samb.—infants, for
11. Pneumonia—Right lung, liver, at the IInd stage or hepatization. Raising mouthful of mucous doesn't give relief. Breath short, nose expands with a fanlike motion. Extreme dyspnoea (Lyc. does wonders-Nash-63). Greyish yellow purulent, salty matter,

much rattling to chest, Lyc.++ indispensable < 4-8 PM, General (4-9 PM of abdominal pain-Coloc.) 4-8 PM Headache+ coryza-Hell. n., Sul., Kali hydro., Sil.

12. Failing Brain power in old people.
    Lyc.+++ Depression, his stupid eyes don't react to light, jaw drops, impending paralysis of Brain.
    Anac.,
    Phos.,
    Baryt. c..,
    Op.,
    Pic. ac.,
    Agn. cast.

VII. Black Letter Symptoms
(Tyler-516-519)

- Mentals, Dread of men; of solitude; irritable and melancholy.
- Weeps all day, cannot calm herself, worse 4 to 8 PM.
- Sensitive: even cries when thanked.
- Satiety of life; particularly mornings in bed.
- Amativeness and amorousness.
- Sensitive, irritable; peevish and cross on waking, Easily excited to anger; cannot bear opposition and is speedily beside herself.
- Ailments from fright, anger, mortification or vexation, with reserved displeasure.
- Oversensitive to pain, Patient is beside herself. (Cham.).
- Speaks wrong words and syllables, selects wrong words.
- Becomes confused about everyday things.
- Great apprehensiveness in the pit of the stomach, (Kali c.).
- Head, Vertigo in the morning when and after rising from bed, so that he reels back and forth.
- Throbbing in brain on leaning head back during the day.
- Throbbing headache after every paroxysm of coughing.

- With the cough, shattering in temples and in chest.
- Pain in temples as if screwed together, worse during menses.
- Rush of blood to head on walking.
- Excessive falling of hair; becomes grey too soon.
- Eyes, distressing pain, as if dry, with nightly, agglutination.
- Styes on lids, more towards inner canthi.
- Ulceration and redness of eyelids.
- Evening light blinds him very much: cannot see anything on the table.
- Roaring, humming, rushing, etc, in Ears.
- Loss of hearing in connection with otorrhoea.
- Eczema of ears, with thick crusts and Fissure.
- Violent catarrh, with swelling of NOSE.
- Stopped catarrh, so that he cannot get breath at night.
- Complete stoppage of nose: child's breath stopped during sleep frequently for fifteen seconds, even while the mouth is open.
- Fan-like motion of the alae nasi.
- FACE yellowish grey.
- Spasmodic twitching of facial muscles.
- TEETH painful when chewing and when touched.
- Numerous blisters on the tongue, Ulcers on and under tongue.
- Feeling as if a ball rose, from below, up into the THROAT.
- Throat feels too tight on swallowing; nothing goes down; food and drink regurgitate through the nose (Gels., Diphth.)
- Excessive appetite, followed by distension of abdomen.
- Hunger remains immediately after eating, though the Stomach and abdomen are full and tense.
- She can't eat at all: is constantly satiated and without appetite: whatever she eats goes against her, even to vomiting.
- Sudden satiety and great thirst.
- Immediately after a meal, is full, bloated, distended.

- Loss of appetite at first mouthful: weight in stomach after eating.
- A sour eructation, the taste does not remain in mouth: but acid gnaws in the stomach.
- Incomplete burning Eructation, which only rise to the pharynx where they cause burning, fir several hours.
- Epigastrium extremely sensitive to touch and tight clothing.
- Digestion seems to proceed very slowly.
- Discomfort in the stomach after eating a little.
- Cramp in the stomach which is much distended.
- Pressure in stomach, as if she had eaten too much.
- Pressure in stomach, as if over-distended, in the evening, after eating a little.
- Pressure, heaviness in stomach, after eating a little in the afternoon.
- Pain in epigastrium caused by coughing.
- She dares not eat to satiety, because if she does, she has an unpleasant, distressed feeling in HEPATIC REGION.
- Pressive pain, hepatic region on breathing.
- Sore pressive pain as from a blow in right hypochondriac region aggravated by touch.
- Liver is painful to touch.
- Pain in left hypochondriac region, afternoon.
- Violent gall-stone colic.
- Ascites from liver affections, after abuse of alcohol.
- Something heavy felt lying in left ABDOMEN not affecting the breathing, but constantly felt while walking, sitting and lying.
- Distension of the abdomen from gases, relieved by emission of flatus.
- Grunting and gurgling in abdomen.
- Whole abdomen distended by flatulence after a stool.
- Much flatus accumulates here and there in abdomen, in hypochondria, even in the back in region of ribs and chest, causing tension and bubbling, always relieved by empty Eructation.

- Immediately after eating the abdomen is constantly full, distended and tense. Tension with incarceration of flatus.
- Sensation of something moving up and down in stomach and bowels, (Comp., Croc., Thuj., Sanic.)
- Hernia right side.
- ANUS painfully closed.
- The rectum so frequently contracted that it protrudes during a hard stool.
- Haemorrhoids painful to touch.
- Great tendency to excoriation about anus; bleed easily. Itching and moist, tender eruption.
- First part of stool lumpy, the second soft.
- Aching in KIDNEY before and after urination.
- Some red sediment in urine.
- Red or reddish yellow sand in urine.
- Turbid, milky urine, with offensive purulent sediment, disposition to calculi.
- Renal colic, particularly right ureter to bladder.
- Urging to urinate; must wait long before it will pass, or inability with constant bearing down. Supports abdomen with hands.
- Night COUGH affecting stomach and diaphragm, mostly before sunset.
- Cough overpowering, evening before going to sleep, as if larynx tickled with a feather, with scanty expectoration.
- Tickling cough as from sulphur fumes larynx.
- Difficult breathing, as if he had inhaled sulphur fumes.
- Grey, salt-tasting expectoration.
- Dyspnoea during sleep; from every exertion.
- CHEST feels oppressed and raw internally.
- Stitches left chest, and during inspiration.
- Hoering gives "Hydro pericardium" (Ars.)
- BACK, burning as from glowing coals between the scapulae (Phos., Kali bich. etc.).
- Severe backache, better by passing urine.
- One foot hot the other cold.
- Desire to go into the open air, (Puls., etc.).

- Her symptoms are aggravated at 4 pm; at 8 PM she feels better but weak.
- Headache, cough, fever, chill, EVERYTHING WORSE 4-8 PM.
- Nervous excitement; prostration of mind and body, Nervous debility.
- Hungry WHEN WAKING; at night.
- On walking, cross, kicks, scolds; un-refreshed.

MAGNESIA CARBONICA

I. Introduction (Cow.-478)

Common Name: Carbonate of Magnesia.
Preparation: Trinturation.
It was proved by Hahnemann. (Pierce-578)

II. General Analysis (Cow.)

Acts upon mucous membrane of the intestinal canal, upon female generative organs, producing irritation and catarrhal inflammation, and deranged menstruation.

III. Suited to (Allen-175)

Persons, especially children of irritable disposition, nervous temperament (Cham.), lax fibre, sour small of whole body (Rhe.).

IV. Clinical (Clarke-II-355)

Antrum of Highmore-disease of, Ascarides, Catarrh, Constipation, Cornea-opacity of, Cough, Deafness, Debility, Diarrhoea, Dyspepsia, Eyes inflamed, Hernia, Menorrhagia, Menstruation delayed, Metrorrhagia, Nervousness, Neuralgia, Neurasthenia, Pregnancy-nausea of; toothache of, Spleen-pain in, Taste disordered, Tinnitus, Toothache, Tumours.

V. Symptoms-General (Nash-337)

1. Stools green, frothy like the scum of frog pond; doubling up colic, > after stool.
2. Toothache in decayed teeth, worse at night, must get up and walk about for relief (especially during pregnancy).
3. Exhausted nerves in worn out women—what China is for loss of blood.

4. Menses; flow only at night or when lying and in absence of uterine pains.

VI. Symptoms-Particular (Nash-337)

Colic.— Mage = Colic

Mag. c.—green frothy stools, preceded by griping double up colic.

Rhe.—Dark brownish sour stools and seems smell of whole body.

Mag. c.—green stool stands first, while with Rheum-Sourness.

Cham.—Green stool with pain but watery.

Merc. c.—Slimy stool may be green with tenesmus.

1. Toothache.

   Mag. c.—in decayed tooth < night <quiet > gentle walk.

   Ratan.—of pregnant women.

2. Menses flow night-Mag. c., Arn. m.
3. Lobel.—extremely sensitive to touch.

MAGNESIA MURIATICA

I. Introduction (Cow.-480)

Synonym: Magnesia chloride.
Common Name: Muriate of Magnesia.
Preparation: Trituration.
It was proved by Hahnemann (Pierce-581).

II. General Analysis (Cow.)

It was proved by Hahnemann who noticed different action of Mag. m. and Mag. c. upon intestinal canal, upon ganglionic nervous system and local influence upon mucous membrane. Constipation. [Difference between Mag. c. and Mag. m. is that the former has diarrhoea and latter constipation as a rule.(Pierce-581)].

III. Suited to (Allen-177)

Especially to the diseases of women—spasmodic and hysterical complaints, complicated with uterine disease, who have suffered for years of indigestion or biliousness. Unable to digest milk. Stool hard, scanty, large, knotty, crumble at verge of anus (Amm. mur., Nat. m.).

IV. Clinical (Clarke-II-364)

Biliousness, Bladder-paresis of, Cardialgia, Colds, Constipation, Deafness, Diarrhoea, Dysmenorrhoea, Dyspepsia, Foot-sweat, Headache, Heart affections, Haemorrhoids, Heartburn, Homesickness, Hysteria, Leucorrhoea, Liver-affections of, Menstruation painful, Nocturnal emissions, Ozaena, Palpitation, Pregnancy-nausea of, Smell disordered, Spleen enlarged, Stomach disordered, Taste disordered, Tinea ciliaris, Urine-straining to pass, Uterus-pain in; induration of, Water-brash, Whooping-cough.

V. Symptoms-General (Nash-338)

1. Constipation; stools knotty or lumpy like sheep dung; crumbling at the verge of the anus.
2. Nervous headache > from pressure (Puls.); on wrapping the head up warmly (Sil.)
3. Palpitation of heart when the patient is quiet, > when moving about.
4. Urine; pale yellow; can only be passed by bearing down with abdominal muscles; weakness of bladder.
5. Adapted to nervous, hysterical women inclined to spasms.

VI. Symptoms-Particular (Nash-339-340)

1. Constipation-Stool like sheep dung, crumble at the verge of anus.
   Amm. mur.,
   Nat. m.
2. Menses painful with sever cramp and spasm with sheep dung stool constipation.
   Amm. mur.
   Mag. c. } menstrual flow is < night.
3. Nervous Headache better from pressure, often hysterical.
   Puls.
   Mag. m. } -strong pressure.
   Sil.-> wrapping head warmly.
4. Spasm with uterine trouble.
   Act. rac.,
   Caul.
5. Liver Troubles.
   Mag. m., } tongue takes imprint of the teeth.
   Merc. s. } < lying on the right side.
   Ptelea.- < when lying on left side.
6. Child doesn't digest milk during dentition.
   Mag. m.,
   Sep.
7. Palpitation of heart.
   < When lying quiet.
   > When moving about.

MAGNESIA PHOSPHORICA

I. Introduction (Clarke-II-369)

Synonym: Phosphate of Magnesia.
Preparation: Trituration.
Mag. phos. was first introduced by Schussler as one of his 12 remedies (Pierce-582).

II. Suited to (Allen-178)

Thin, emaciated persons of a highly nervous organisation, dark complexioned. Affection of right side of body (Bell., Bry., Chel., Kali c., Lyc., Podo.) Pains-crampy in neuralgic affections of stomach, Dread of uncovering, of cold air. Headache—begins in occiput to head (Sang., Sil.) > pressure and external heat.

III. Clinical (Clarke-II-369)

Catheterism, Chorea, Colic, Convulsions, Cough, Cracks, Cramps, Dentition, Dysmenorrhoea, Headache, Intercostal neuralgia, Locomotor ataxy, Membranous dysmenorrhoea, Meningitis, Menstruation painful, Neuralgia, Rectum-prolapse of, School-headache, Sciatica, Stomach-cancer of, Sobbing-spasmodic, Tic douloureux, Toothache, Vaginismus, Whooping-cough, Writer's cramp.

IV. Symptoms-General (Nash-340)

1. Cramping pains everywhere, also lightning-like in coming and going.
2. Spasmodic affections without febrile symptoms. Colic, whooping-cough, cramp in calves, etc.
3. Modalities: < cold water, touch, > heat warmth, pressure, bending double.

V. Symptoms-Particular (Nash 340-341)

1. Mag. phos. is amongst "very best neuralgia or pain remedies".
2. Cramping pains, often changing place.
   (mostly-in stomach, abdomen, pelvis).
3. Colic of infants.
   Mag. phos.,
   Cham.,
   Coloc.
4. Dysmenorrhea, neuralgic with crampy pains.
   Mag. phos.—Best medicine.
5. Relief from hot application—is most pronounced in Mag. phos. (Ars.).
   Mag. phos.—Various kind of pains except burning pains.
   Ars.-Burning pain > Hot.
6. Painful Menstruation.
   Mag. phos. is quicker than Puls., Caul., Cimicif. r.
   Pain ceases when flow begins.

7. Pains.
   -Cramping—Cupr., Coloc., Mag. phos.
   -Burning—Ars., Canth., Caps., Phos., Sul. a.
   -Coldness (Sensation)—Calc. c., Ars., Helod., Cistus.
   -Coldness (Objective)—Camph., Sec., Verat., Helod.
   -Fullness-(Sensation)—Æsc. hip., China, Lyc.
   -Emptiness (Sensation)—Coca, Phos., Sep.
   -Bearing down—Bell., Lil. t., Sep.
   -Bruised soreness—Arn., Bap., Eup. perf., Rut., Pyr.
   -Constriction—Cact., Coloc., Anac.
   -Prostration—Gels., Pic. ac., Phos. ac.
   -Numbness—Acon., Plat., Rhus t., Cham.
   -Erratic pain—Lac can., Puls., Tuberc.
   -Sensitive to pain—Acon., Coff., Cham.
   -Sensitive to touch—China, Hep. s., Lach.
   -Bone pains—Aur. m., Asa., Eup. perf., Merc. c.
   -Stitching sticking pains—Bry., Kali c., Squil.
   -Throbbing—Bell., Glon., Meli.

-Haemorrhage (Passive)—Ham., Sec., Crotal. h., Elap.
-Haemorrhage (Active)—Ferr. phos., Ipec., Phos.
-Emaciation—Iod., Nat. m., Lyc., Sarsa.
-Leucophlegmasia—Calc. c., Graph., Caps.
-Constitution (Psoric)—Sul., Psor., Graph., Caust., etc.
-Constitution (Sycotic)—Thuj., Nit. ac., Medo., etc.
-Constitution (Syphilitic)—Merc. i. fl., Syph., etc.
-Blue swelling—Lach., Puls., Tarent. cub.

VI. Black Letter Symptoms
(Tyler-524-525)

- Neuralgia or rheumatic headache; better from external application of warmth: very excruciating.
- Tendency to spasmodic symptoms.
- Shooting, stinging, shifting, intermittent or spasmodic pains: sparks before the eyes.
- More in young and strong persons. After mental labour.
- Neuralgic pain, especially behind right ear: worse by going into cold air, and washing face and neck in cold water.
- Otalgia, purely nervous.
- Toothache, better by heat and hot lids.
- Severe pain in decayed or filled teeth: swelling of tongue.
- Complaints of teething children.
- Spasms during dentition, no fever.
- Spasms or cramp in stomach, nipping, griping, pinching, with short belching of wind, giving no relief.
- Spasms or cramp in stomach, with clean tongue: as if a hand was tightly laced or drawn round body.
- Enteralgia.
- Flatulent colic forcing patient to bend double: (Coloc.) better from rubbing, warmth, pressure. Accompanied by belching of gas, which gives no relief.
- Bloated, full sensation in abdomen; must loosen clothes (Lyc.) and walk about.

- Flatulent colic of children and the new born, with drawing up of legs: remittent colic; crampy pain with acidity.
- Radiating pain in abdomen.
- Meteorism in cows (Colch.).
- Nocturnal enuresis from nervous irritation.
- Menstrual Colic.
- Membranous dysmenorrhoea.
- Ovarian neuralgia, pain shooting and darting like lightning worse on the right side.
- Spasmodic, nervous asthma.
- Chorea.
- Neuralgia at intervals, relieved by warmth.
- Chilliness: chills run up and down the back (Gels.) with shivering.
- Dread of uncovering (Nux. v.).
- Worse: right side; from cold; from touch: relieved by warmth; by beding double.

MEDORRHINUM

I. Introduction (Clarke-II-409)

Synonym: Glinicum
Common Name: Nosode of Gonorrhoea
Preparation: Attenuations of the virus.

II. Suited to (Allen-180)

Bad effects of maltreatment and suppression of gonorrhoea, when best selected remedies fail to cure. Ailments: which can be traced to psychotic origin; gout, rheumatism, neuralgia, and diseases of spinal cord and its membranes. Women with or without psychotic origin, overites, pelvic cellulitis, fibroids, cysts and other morbid growth of uterus and ovaries. Same relation to deep seated psychotic chronic affections of spinal cord and sympathetic system which Psorinum has to deep seated skin and mucous membrane affections. State of collapse (Carb. v.—skin cold yet throws covers, opp. of Nux. v.) cold perspiration (Verat.). < from daylight to sunset (Reverse of Syph.).

III. Clinical (Clarke-II-409)

Asthma, Clonic spasms, Corns, Diabetes, Dysmenorrhoea, Epilepsy, Eyes inflamed, Favus, Gleet, Gonorrhoea-suppressed, Gonorrhoeal rheumatism, Headache-neuralgic, Liver-abscess of, Masturbation, Ovaries-pain in, Pelvic cellulitis, Polypi, Priapism, Psoriasis palmaris, Ptosis, Renal colic, Rheumatism, Sciatica, Shoulder-pains in, Stricture, Urticaria, Warts.

IV. Symptoms-Particular (Nash-423)

1. Chronic Rheumatism—ankle joints stiff, soles tender, unable to walk.
   Medo.,
   Ant. c.—when it does not improve.

2. Nightly bone pains (including spinal).
   Syph.—When of syphilitic origin < Night.
   Medo.—when otherwise < day time.

V. Black Letter Symptoms

(Tyler-534-535)

- Time moves too slowly.
- Dullness of memory ; desire to procrastinate, because business seemed so lasting, or as if it could never be accomplished.
- In conversation would stop, and remark he could not think what word wanted to use.
- Fears he is going to die.
- Is in a great hurry: in such a hurry that he feels fatigued.
- Epistaxis.
- Continuous watering of eyes: sensation of sand under lids.
- Impotence.
- Incipient consumption.
- Great pallor; yellowness of face, particularly around eyes, as if from a bruise. Yellow band across forehead close to hair.
- Neuralgia right upper and lower jaws, extending to temple.
- Hard swelling right upper jaw, as if in socket of a tooth gone years ago.
- Pale gums.
- Very sore mouth; ulcers on tongue and in mouth, like blisters.
- Blisters inner surface cheeks and lips; skin peeling in patches.
- Violent retching and vomiting for forty-eight hours, first glairy mucous, lastly coffee grounds, with intense headache, great despondency and sensation of impending death: during paroxysm was constantly praying.
- Cramp in stomach as from wind.
- Sensation in pit of stomach as of a paper of pins, that seemed to force themselves through the flesh, causing her to rise and double up and scream: pins seem to come from each side.

- Intense pain in stomach and upper abdomen, with sensation of tightness.
- Congestion of liver.
- Burning heat round back like a coal of fire.
- Throbbing—a thumping in region of suprarenal capsule, as if from abscess or sore spot just below fifth rib, right side, creeping chills in region of right kidney, throbbing, contracting, drawing and relax as if caused by cold insects with claws.
- Ascites: abdomen greatly distended, urine scanty and kigh coloured.
- Black stool.
- White diarrhoea.
- Can only pass stool by leaning far back; very painful; as if a lump on posterior surface of sphincter, so painful as to cause tears.
- Cholera infantum with opisthotonos, vomiting and watery diarrhoea: profuse discharge of blood and pus.
- Painful attacks of piles, nor bleeding; swelling left anus.
- Pin worms.